FEWER

FEWER

*How the New Demography of Depopulation
Will Shape Our Future*

Ben J. Wattenberg

Ivan R. Dee
CHICAGO 2004

The paperback edition of this book carries the ISBN 1-56663-673-6.

Library of Congress Cataloging-in-Publication Data:
Wattenberg, Ben J.
    Fewer : how the new demography of depopulation will shape our future / Ben J. Wattenberg.
        p. cm.
    Includes bibliographical references and
    index. ISBN: 978-1-56663-673-5

    1. Population. 2. Fertility, Human. I. Title.
HB871.W35 2004
304.6'2--dc22

2004050016

To my grandchildren, Emma, Michael, and Lylah

Contents

FEWER

Part One

WHAT HAPPENED
AND WHY?

CHAPTER ONE

The Story of This Book

THIS BOOK is about demography, that is, the study of populations, that is, human beings, that is, people.

For at least 650 years, since the time of the Black Plague, the total number of people on earth has headed in only one direction: *up*. But soon—probably within a few decades—global population will level off and then likely fall for a protracted period of time. The number of people on earth will be headed *down*, "depopulating."

Why? Birthrates and fertility rates ultimately yield total population levels. *And never have birth and fertility rates fallen so far, so fast, so low, for so long, in so many places, so surprisingly.*

Depopulation is already proceeding in many of the modern developed nations. Europe is now losing about 700,000 people each year, a figure that will grow to about 3 million a year, or more, by midcentury. Russia alone is losing close to a million people each year. Within the next few years Japan will begin losing population. The steep trend toward fewer children per woman in the modern nations has been near universal. Only the United States is an exception, one which will be discussed in many places in this book. These trends may have an intense personal relevance for many Americans.

But what's going on is not restricted to the well-to-do modern nations. The poorer, Less Developed Countries (LDCs), still have higher birth and fertility rates than the rich countries. But rates in the LDCs are typically falling at a more rapid rate than ever experienced in the rich countries. As recently as 1970 the typical woman in an LDC

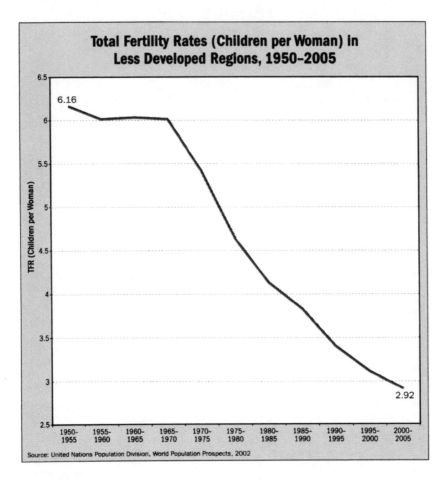

Total Fertility Rates (Children per Woman) in Less Developed Regions, 1950–2005

Source: United Nations Population Division, World Population Prospects, 2002

nation bore 6.0 children per woman. Today, in the midst of a fertility free-fall, the rate is about 2.8 or 2.7 children per woman and rapidly continuing downward. Such patterns have been observed in India, Indonesia, Brazil, Egypt, Iran, and, critically, Mexico, only to begin a long list. This is not idle speculation. These are not simple straight-line projections. As we shall see, much of it is already pretty well baked into the cake of the future, baked into the New Demography.

Why the continuing decline? One example: Billions of people still live in rural poverty. They are migrating to cities, where fertility and family size are invariably lower than in rural areas. The results are already inscribed in official United Nations projections. Moreover, I believe the UN is most likely understating the actual speed of the current fertility decline.

The New Demography is here. It relates to most everything involved in human activity, and its consequences can only intensify. What is happening will affect parents, grandparents, and children everywhere. It will affect every business in every country. After all, the numbers of customers, or lack thereof, is at the essence of commerce and economics, of buying and selling. Population is at the center of our environmental situation. This includes the air we breathe, the water we drink, and perhaps the level at which we set the thermostat. It relates to traffic jams. It relates to what is often called suburban sprawl, or the absence of it. Population holds a fine mirror to many human values and how they change.

Even before 9/11, and certainly since then, the New Demography has had a great impact on geopolitics—the high-stakes games that nations play. The United States is now called "the sole superpower." It also has a unique demographic signature: America will grow while all the other modern nations will shrink. What will America be then? The only omnipower? Or a muscle-bound polyglot, a bickering and overextended giant player on the global scene, harming itself and others?

After 9/11, as I worked on this book, I watched television, read the newspapers and magazines, went to seminars, interviewed experts. Something was missing. President Bush said we have to save our civilization. If you are engaged in speculating about how to save civilization, demography is an important dimension, indeed a critical one. But I had the feeling that most commentators don't know demography from pornography. Even some expert demographers have no idea of how rapidly things have changed.

The New Demography may well intensify the cry that America is "going it alone"—not because we want to, but rather because we have to. Our principal allies, the people in Europe and Japan, are bearing almost unbelievably few children.

How will it all turn out? The best may yet to be, with America in the lead. Alternatively, America's demographic wave may crash on the sharp rocks of immigration and separatism, other aspects of the current demographic situation. And as America goes, so goes the world. (For the record, early on, I think it will work out pretty well.) The starkest aspects of the new global demographic era I write about will probably be of limited duration, most likely playing themselves out in the course of this century. Many readers will likely see much of the process in their lifetimes.

Demography is a curious field of study. Everyone knows that population is important, but if I asked you to name a famous demographer, you'd probably say, "I don't know," or "Malthus." And what about Malthus? Two hundred years ago he wrote his famous essay explaining that population growth would outpace food supply, causing famine and tragedy. He was wrong, and acknowledged it.

It is often said that "demography is destiny." That's an overstatement, but it's nonetheless crucial. If we are aware of the accelerating trends, we may want to try to shape our demography and consequently help shape our destiny. As a general matter, not many people are aware of what's going on, including the high and mighty in the policy community.

The advent of the New Demography portends a different world. Joseph Chamie, director of the UN Population Division (UNPD), puts it this way: There was the Industrial Revolution. There was The Information Age. Now there is the Demographic Revolution.

At root the situation is fairly simple: the numbers of people on earth will grow by an ever-diminishing rate, level off, then begin shrinking. World population now numbers about six billion. That number will grow to eight to nine billion, depending on whose numbers you accept. Then population will decrease, perhaps by many billions. What is not so simple is how life plays out as this happens— who does it help and who does it hurt; why is it happening; can we do anything about it, should we, and if so, what.

I try to avoid technical terms and a waterfall of charts and statistics in this book, but some are necessary and they are here.

This book has an unusual history. In 1987 I wrote *The Birth Dearth*, in which I looked at the "Total Fertility Rate." Simply put, the TFR represents the average number of children born per woman over the course of her childbearing years. If the average woman in a given country bears three children, the TFR for that country is 3.0.* The

---

*Why is the TFR counted by the number of children per woman, not man? Two reasons: when a woman has a baby, the mother knows it; and a woman's reproductive life is shorter.

TFR is the keystone calculation of demography, and I would argue that it is the single most important measurement of humankind. Moreover, it comes with some precision.

After all, economic projections and predictions can change on a dime when Thailand's currency hits a wall or an "Asian Contagion" roils the markets. Political science is an oxymoron, as many practitioners will cheerfully admit. (In the spring of 1992, during the Democratic primary elections, many political scholars and pundits explained why candidate Bill Clinton was "toast.") But demography has much more predictive value. Demographers can tell you in 2004 with some certainty how many twenty-year-old potential mothers there will be in 2025.

How so? Because those potential mothers of the future would already have been born twenty years ago. They have been counted by censuses in most all areas of the world and put in a statistical "cohort," that is, the number of persons in a given age group, say, from age zero to age ten. Then—surprise!—every twelve months, like clockwork, the surviving members of the cohort are one year older. The deaths of infants and children who never reach their own age of reproduction are then factored into the equation.

Alas, we do not know everything about those twenty-year-old potential mothers. We know roughly how many there will be in 2025, but we don't know how many children they will decide to bear. In the poor countries they may have 3.0 children per woman, or perhaps only 2.0, or less. Still, we do know something fairly definite about the future, and that is not to be gainsaid.

By the mid-1980s, when I wrote *The Birth Dearth,* something quite remarkable was already happening in the demographic arena. Women in the "modern" countries were bearing substantially fewer children than are required to "replace" a population—that is, fewer children than would be needed just to keep a population at a stable level over an extended time (not counting net gain or loss from immigration or increased or decreased longevity).

The "replacement" level in modern countries is a Total Fertility Rate of 2.1 children per woman. That is the so-called "magic number" in demography. Why 2.1? Sooner or later a mother and father die. If the parents are not "replaced" by two children—plus one-tenth of a child to account for those children who do not live to reach their own age of reproduction—over time the population declines. (There are other factors as well.)

When I wrote *The Birth Dearth*, the average Total Fertility Rate in the "Developed Regions," as the UN labels modern countries, had sunk to 1.8 children per woman. The rate was about the same in the United States. That number was about 14 percent below the 2.1 replacement value. But there was something else: the TFR in the Developed Regions had been falling steadily for *thirty-five years*. This was no short-term trend.

That level of births for a large group of nations was the lowest ever recorded, except during times of temporary catastrophe. This trend would affect commerce. It would affect pensions. It had vast environmental implications. It might affect the geopolitical balance of power and influence. It was ignored.

But *The Birth Dearth* was not ignored. The book attracted a great deal of attention, positive and negative. Steve Forbes, in his eponymous magazine, wrote, "Here is a book that will join the ranks of Rachel Carson's *Silent Spring*." I liked that, but, alas, it was not to be.

Some of the negative comments about *The Birth Dearth* indicated that I might be a sexist, a cold warrior, a racist, a polluter, and, worst, a straight-linist. (Demographers correctly like to emphasize that projections aren't predictions. I believe I was just following the data.) Even one of the most influential men in world history, Paul Ehrlich, the author of the *The Population Bomb*, deigned to weigh in on one of his many fields of expertise: the demographic aspects of military policy. There was no link, he wrote, between population size and military power, asking: "How many able-bodied, healthy young men are required to push a few buttons?" (Answer: In America, about $450 billion worth of defense spending each year, coming from the taxes of about 300 million people.) As we shall see, straightforward demographic numbers can engender mighty arguments.

I fought my fight on this matter and moved on. But during the late 1980s and through the 1990s I kept half an eye cocked to the emerging demographic picture. Periodically I wrote a column on demographic matters. I enjoyed it; the topic has been my first and most enduring love as a writer. (Too much of our politics repeats itself and becomes routine; demography in our era has been kaleidoscopic.)

As the century closed and millennial fever mounted, I decided to adopt a new dimension to my personal regimen of the study of demography. Every thousand years, I vowed, I would look with fresh eyes at the new edition of my favorite book, the UN's biennial *World Population Prospects*.* To the uninitiated it is a huge scramble of numbers. For demographers, and for demographic hangers-on like me, it is the bedrock of the field, containing an array of data from the 192 largest nations and areas (those with populations of over 100,000 people). Based on the data, it presents four different population projections for each nation: "high," "medium," "low," and "constant-fertility variant."

In early 2001, when I scanned the new 2000 edition, I was wide-eyed. This was no plain vanilla birth dearth. The bottom had fallen out.

First, the already low European and Japanese rates were sinking with dizzying speed. The 1.8 children per woman of the 1980s were projected at 1.3 children per woman in the 2000–2005 time frame—that's now. Repeat: from 1.8 to 1.3 in a single generation. That 1.3 European rate is 38 percent below the replacement level. That level is unheard-of, previously unimaginable. No serious demographer would plausibly have predicted such a sharp decline even a decade earlier.

But most Europeans seemed to yawn at this news. After all, for decades the bedrock UN demographic projection had been stating that over the course of the next half-century or so the European and Japanese TFRs would likely drift back upward to the 2.1 replacement level. This projection was based on absolutely no evidence. Nor would a projected population rebound likely come from massive immigration. By American standards, the European countries had taken in only moderate numbers of immigrants, mostly Muslims—and for the most part typically abhorred what they had done, or what had been done to them.

World Population Prospects is available for $80 at the UN bookstore at UN headquarters in New York City. The price is steep, but nearly all the findings are available free of charge on the internet at unpopulation.org. A CD-ROM is available for $800; poor nations get one free.

The principal rationale of the UN Population Division seemed to be, "These kinds of low and lower rates in Europe can't continue or these countries will go out of business." The UN demographic record-keepers treated the Japanese in roughly the same manner— that is, they projected a resurgence from 1.3 to about 2.1 children per woman by the mid-twenty-first century. (And the Japanese despise immigrants, probably even more so than do the Europeans.)

The second eye-opener from *World Population Prospects* was that a major abnormality seemed to be taking shape. While the fertility rate in the modern nations fell sharply, in the United States the rate moved up—not quite to the replacement level, but up. How long it will stay up remains to be seen, and we should be careful in thinking about it. But for now America is quite clearly the most baby-making of the world's major modern nations. Moreover, Americans take in a solid number of immigrants, higher by far than do the Europeans or Japanese. One estimate has it that America takes in as many legal immigrants as the entire rest of the world together.

Thus the United States, principally because of immigration, was growing steadily and would continue to do so. The UN medium variant projection called for about 400 million Americans by the year 2050, up from 283 million in 2000. (The first U.S. Census, taken in 1790, showed 3.9 million people.) As I saw it, through my much-worn magenta lenses, this was yet further evidence that America should be seen as the world's most exceptional nation, with much of human destiny resting on its shoulders.

And even that wasn't the biggest part of the story. Another potent trend, apparent in that 2000 volume, was becoming ever more evident. Many people interested in public affairs have an inchoate notion about low fertility rates, though they may have a small sense of the recent magnitude of the Euro-Japanese decline. But of the recent demographic trends in motion in the nonmodern countries, those that used to be called "Third World," there is almost total ignorance. Most anyone will tell you that population is "exploding" in these places. Indeed, I had dealt with this in *The Birth Dearth* but in the context of the upside, not the downside. The TFR for all the Less Developed Countries had dropped from six children in the first half of the 1960s to about four children in the early 1980s. That's a big drop. It was encouraging; I duly noted it would continue downward. But four children per woman is still far above replacement level and would yield nothing but substantially more population in those poorer countries, for a long time.

This was the powerful message stressed at various points on the political spectrum. Notwithstanding very low fertility in the modern countries, notwithstanding forthcoming European and Japanese depopulation, the total *world* population would grow substantially for several decades, gobbling up resources, polluting the planet, warming the climate, forcing unwanted immigration on the modern nations, and, always lurking in the background, changing the balance of power while altering patterns of race, culture, and ethnicity in the world. It was implied that the human species could run out of control, that the world might even find many species disappearing as rapacious humans built ever more fast-food joints in the middle of the rain forests. In truth, there was some real merit in what environmentalists had to say—along with a heavy dose of demographic demagoguery—during this remarkable run of population growth. A quadrupling of global population in a single century was something to write home about.

But so dramatic was the new data from the late 1980s and the 1990s that what was happening in the Less Developed Countries now had to be seen in a different way. It was very much a part of the forthcoming depopulation process rather than an exception to it.

As shown in an earlier chart, the TFR for the Less Developed Countries had fallen to 2.9 children per woman, from a high of 6 children in the late 1960s, a drop of more than three children per woman. The rate had dropped by 52 percent, but that's misleading. More important, it had dropped about 85 percent of the way toward replacement-level fertility!

The end of worldwide population growth was thus clearly in sight, albeit through midrange lenses. And not one person in a thousand, if that, had a clue about it. It was pretty clear to me, and many demographers, that the number of children per woman would keep on falling rapidly, for reasons I will explain. Then, quite possibly before midcentury, total world population itself would then begin to fall. Who could envision a world where India, Bangladesh, Brazil, Mexico, the Muslim countries, and the even poorer sub-Saharan African countries would lose population from natural decline?

Then, in March 2002—after publication of the UN's 2000 *Revisions* volume but before publication of its 2002 volume (which appeared in early 2003)—the UN officially revised its thinking on a very important matter. Its scholarly Population Division announced that new and different projections were on the way, whose implications would be nothing less than "momentous." This is not the way scholars normally talk to one another. It was high praise of oneself from oneself, and in this case it was fully merited.

I date the advent of the New Demography from that moment. After decades of dillydallying, the UN Population Division bit the bullet. Finally the world's official source showed as its medium projection that the Less Developed Countries would emulate the more developed nations and fall below the replacement level. Then, according to the UN, world population would decline in the latter part of the twenty-first century. Yes, decline, in this century. I think it will happen sooner, within three to four decades, perhaps a bit longer. I will offer reasons.

I was invited to be a participant in a UN conference of demographers to discuss the matter, as I had been once before. I was amazed by what I heard. As the lights blinked in the simultaneous translation booths and demographers seated around a long oval table sipped their coffee, a bare-bones story took on meat. The demographer from Iran reported that the TFR in his officially Less Developed Country, a despotic Islamic theocracy, a charter member of the "Axis of Evil"—had already fallen to 2.06 children per woman, that is, below the replacement level. A demographer from Brazil spoke in Spanish because there were no Portuguese interpreters available. She said that Brazil was already likely below replacement level and that the UN hadn't quite caught up with reality.

And then another shocker. The Mexican demographer said that her country would fall below the replacement level by 2005. If so, what about the tan tide of humanity surging up across the Rio Grande that had so traumatized Pat Buchanan and many other Americans? In years to come, if Mexico fell below replacement level and

Mexicans, legal and illegal, continued coming to America, wouldn't Mexico empty out?

And that wasn't all. Suddenly, most all the other demographic shibboleths were under question. Stone-faced, the professional social scientists noted that something more than the correlations of the past was under way. The old ones had seen the relationships between the education of women and low fertility, between numbers of working women and low fertility, between government family-planning programs and low fertility. Now something new was happening. Around me at the table were experts who had been caught with their correlations down, acknowledging that the roots of their discipline were planted in wet sand. They knew what was happening, but they did not know why.

All this is not as technical as it may seem. I am not a demographer, though I am an admirer of demographers. I look at their output. (You can too; go to the web.) Simply put, the UN had announced that henceforward it would assume that average fertility in the poor countries would fall not just to 2.1 children per woman, as it had rigidly assumed through the 2000 volume. *For the 2002 volume it would fall to 1.85 children per woman.*

All calculations in this book, unless otherwise noted, are based on that 2002 volume. Here is one that arrived after publication of the 2002 volume: South Korea's National Statistical Office announced that its TFR for 2002 was 1.17 children per woman. That was substantially below the 1.41 number reported in the UN's 2002 volume and places South Korea among the lowest TFR nations in the world and the lowest in Asia except for two city-states—Hong Kong, the world's lowest at 1.0 children per woman, and Macao at 1.1 children per woman.

The 2002 differential between 2.1 and 1.85 is significant, a full quarter of a child per woman. But beyond the numbers it is Copernican in the scope of its implications. Copernicus said the earth moves around the sun, not the other way around. Similarly, there is a big difference between a car moving forward at five miles per hour, or a car that is stationary, or a car that is moving backward at five miles per hour. The new UN population estimate said that world population would go down, not up. The car would move backward.

By my lights this data should change the way human beings look at their own species—personally, geopolitically, culturally, economically, and environmentally. I began thinking this might offer something of a challenge to the public perception of Darwinism. Weren't we humans supposed to have been bred for billions of years with a hefty premium on surviving? By definition, a species doesn't survive with an ongoing below-replacement fertility rate.* (No, I don't think the human species will unbreed itself out of existence.)

The drop from 2.1 to 1.85 was big news because it broke a long-standing UN conceit: that every nation would rise or fall near to a Total Fertility Rate of 2.1 children per woman. But concealed beneath the momentous change was a big bet beyond the potency of the 1.85 figure. For example, the UN demographers were saying that the European TFR of 1.38 children per women would climb to 1.85 children per woman (up 34 percent), despite the fact that the European TFR had fallen for *fifty* consecutive years. They were counting on an increase of almost half a child per woman, no small matter. As will be seen later, there is no particular reason to project such a major boost and many reasons to think it will remain low.

I HAD THE UN INFORMATION early and wrote about it for the *Wall Street Journal*, in a piece headlined "Over-population Is Over-hyped." But I had been writing that sort of stuff for decades. More interesting was that two days later a four-column headline appeared in the Sunday *New York Times*: "Population Estimates Fall as Poor Women Assert Control," with a subhead reading: "In India, Brazil, Egypt and Mexico, a Dip in Birthrates Defies Old Theories." A sidebar displayed a graph that showed how the new projections would cut India's estimated population by 85 million people by 2050. By 2150 the reduction in India would be 686 million.

Those 686 million never-born Indians would amount to more than twice the current total population of the United States. Might it be that when the official world body and the official world newspaper announced such a dramatic finding, the world's movers and

---

*Experts in the field of evolutionary psychology have explained to me that what Darwin meant by survival was not what I was talking about, and that the new UN data did not work for or against Darwin's ideas. So be it.

shakers would take notice and start thinking through these events that "defy old theories"? They didn't.

Of course, within the population industry it caused a tidal wave. Since the time of Malthus there has been an apocalyptic cast to the most publicized of demographic findings. In their 1985 book, *The Fear of Population Decline*, Michael Teitelbaum and Jay Winter documented the downside of such history.

Malthus was originally concerned about population increase. Neo-Malthusians in our own time believed in a "population explosion," which would wreak havoc both environmentally and economically. Indeed, global population grew from 1.65 billion to 6.07 billion during the twentieth century. But with the new low-fertility UN data, some alarmists feared that population growth would no longer be regarded as the preeminent problem in the world. Some activists denounced the UN Population Division as turncoats.

The key sentence in the UN's 2002 report is the very last one. It says its findings reveal a demography in motion that "will lead first to a slowing of population growth rates and then to *slow reductions* in the size of world populations" (italics mine). In one sentence, fifty years of demographic study were reversed. I would take issue with only one word: "slow." I think there is a good deal of evidence to show that depopulation will happen rather faster, though these matters are relative. But before things settle, we may find ourselves with quite a few billion fewer people than we thought we'd have.

Still, I salute the United Nations Population Division. It took them too long to break the demographic sound barrier, but it was a major accomplishment. We should all be able to think more clearly now. In coming years I believe the UNPD will take its population and fertility projections even lower.

So I ask some questions here: What's happening? Why? What might it lead to? In the course of dealing with these questions, I ask whether we can or should do something about this shift. Will America remain the demographic exception and shape the twenty-first century? Might America grow so populous that it startles even me?

I was busily working away for a few months about the role of the New Demography when the Twin Towers crashed to earth, when the Pentagon was slammed, and when President George W. Bush said that Americans had been thrust into a war to save our Western civilization. Many agreed, including me.

When I began looking at the great game civilizations play, I studied Samuel Huntington's tour de force, *The Clash of Civilizations*, which maintains that America and the West are on the way down while Islam and the Asian countries are headed for greater glory, in part because of demographic trends. Huntington's book had been published in 1996 but took on substantial new stature in the wake of 9/11. I interviewed him for my weekly PBS television discussion program "Think Tank." He is one smart fellow.

I also read Pat Buchanan's anti-Mexican screed, which throws up the fear of a Latin invasion of America. His book is summed up neatly in its title, *The Death of the West: How Dying Populations and Immigrant Invasion Imperil Our Country and Civilization*. Buchanan had learned something about demographics and spun it into ugly cloth. He also knew a lot about geopolitics, much of it wrongheaded in my view. We had a contentious pair of sessions on "Think Tank."

All this led me down some paths I had not expected to tread upon, which I have worked into my original structure for this book. The United States, the sole superpower, would be growing—but would it remain strong? The vast majority of our immigration was now arriving from non-European nations. Would they assimilate? If they didn't, could a divided America remain assertive on the global stage just when it was most needed? Would we begin limiting immigration? These questions, and others, were brought to mind even more starkly in 2003 after diplomatic action in the UN and military action in Afghanistan and Iraq led by the United States.

As pieces of the U.S. Census of 2000 appeared, one demographic story did crash the headlines: America, it was said, would be mostly "nonwhite" by midcentury. As we shall see, that's not entirely correct. Still, some of the troops of Political Correctitude were demanding that George Washington's picture come down from classroom walls because the man owned slaves. Would we be able, as we once did, to teach American patriotism to American children?

Who wins and who loses in the arc of history we stand astride? Clearly, demographics plays a major role in answering that question.

CHAPTER TWO

And Then There Were Many Fewer

AT FIRST GLANCE it appears that the modern nations of the European landmass are engaged in a process that ends up with a demographic auctioneer saying, "Going, going, gone!" It's not that bad, but still astonishing and, by my lights, disheartening. I hear American commentators, particularly of a conservative bent, say, "Europe is a decadent place. Europeans have never recovered from their loss of empire. Europe's leaders and intellectuals are so snotty to America and the American way of life because they are jealous and increasingly irrelevant." I can only add that if that view were correct, the astonishingly low European fertility numbers would tend to prove the proposition.

In the aggregate, the European nations are known officially in UN demographic data as part of the "Developed Regions." At one time most of these nations were often called the "First World," in distinction to the poor nations of the "Third World," while the command economy nations of the Soviet bloc were sometimes characterized as the "Second World." In the UN Population Division documents the distinction initially was "More Developed Countries" and "Less Developed Countries." Apparently these classifications were seen as somewhat demeaning. How could the United Nations, of all organizations, possibly declare that one nation be less than any other nation, or more? And so the UN classifiers went to work. Today, officially, there are only the unwieldy terms "Developed" nations and "Developing" nations. (I expect the next change will be to "Group A" and "Group B," with "Group B" labeling the rich nations.) I use here the clearer previous terminology, More Developed Countries and Less Developed Countries. Other loose synonyms for the developed nations include "modern" nations, or the "West," or "Western civilization." At various times in this book these terms appear almost interchangeably.

Qualifications for the club include relative affluence, democratic governance in many forms, and general modernity. In this grouping are all the European nations, including Russia all the way out to Siberia (including the nations of Ukraine and Belarus), the North American nations of the United States and Canada, and the Pacific nations of Japan, Australia, and New Zealand. The major plausible exception in this group is Russia, which is not nearly as modern, affluent, or democratic as the others, and certainly not as healthy. But Russia appears to be moving in the right direction, though the headlines seem to change day by day.

The inclusion of Japan is noteworthy. We often say "West" but what we hear, or think, is "white." Japan is not white, nor for that matter is it of the West in any geographic sense. But for almost sixty years it has been a modern, well-to-do, and democratic nation. That puts it in the club, and the UN counts it that way. Thus: most white nations are developed, but all developed nations are not white. About modernity, then, think economics, not biology; think class, not race.

The antecedents of the New Demography among the modern nations are most interesting. In the early 1950s, the decade following the end of World War II, women in the developed nations typically bore 2.7 children over the course of their fertile years. That 2.7 was a high level for a modern nation in the mid-twentieth century. But there were quite clear reasons for at least a part of the elevated rate. In the 1930s the world had experienced the deepest, longest, and most widespread economic depression ever recorded. It was immediately followed by World War II, which, unlike World War I, encompassed most of the planet. Together, the depression and World War II caused many couples to delay their childbearing plans, even to alter

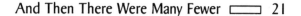

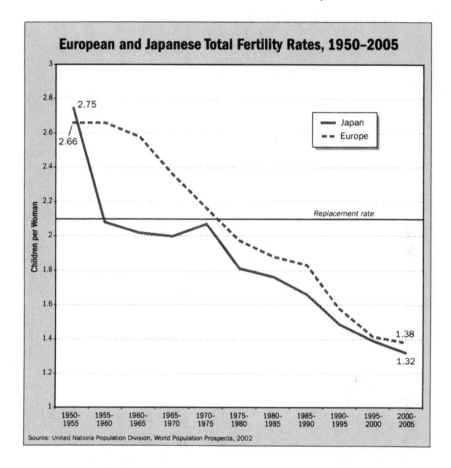

European and Japanese Total Fertility Rates, 1950–2005

Source: United Nations Population Division, World Population Prospects, 2002

their childbearing ability. The depression made it difficult to provide the wherewithal to raise and support children. The war took many potential fathers out of contact with women, and vice versa.

By the mid-1940s both the war and the depression had ended. Spirits rebounded, and so did fertility. Couples "making up for lost time" contributed mightily to the so-called Baby Boom throughout the developed world. In the 1950s in the United States, where the boom was particularly potent and extended, the Total Fertility Rate soared as high as 3.8 children per woman. That rate is far above what today would be described as "Third World" fertility. New American suburbs were nicknamed "Fertile Acres." America was in heat.

The Baby Boom was surely an important story, and one whose results we are still living with. But it bears repeating that at least part of it came about due to extraneous reasons: depression and war. Twenty-five years after the end of World War II (the 1970–1975 time frame), the 1950 TFR of 2.8 children per woman for all the modern nations had already receded to 2.1. That was a 24 percent decline, down to just the rate at which a population remains stable over time.

All seemed in demographic order in the modern world in the early 1970s. The demographic magic number of 2.1 had been reached.

Surely that 2.1 rate or thereabouts is what most demographers had assumed would happen. Most long-term demographic projections, including the most cited of the UN projections, had showed fertility leveling off at 2.1 for both More Developed and Less Developed countries, albeit at very different moments in history. Over the long term, after all, how could it be otherwise? If the TFR dipped substantially below replacement and stayed there, humankind would eventually disappear, proceeding to zero at a steep geometric rate of decline. If it remained above replacement, and stayed there, we would experience a real population explosion, expanding geometrically— the resultant pile of newly born human flesh expanding at the speed of light, which is how one explosionist described the situation to a congressional committee.

The standard graphs were elegant, sloping gracefully to the mystical level of 2.1, where it stayed, apparently forever. One could sense the presence of design in the equation of humanity, perhaps even a divine design.

This elegant formula was part of what experts called the "Demographic Transition," which had been in motion for several hundred years in the modern world. Briefly put, Transition Theory explains how a population moves from high fertility and high mortality and to low fertility and low mortality. It may sound more complicated than it is.

Consider a simple version of Transition Theory. In the old days, before modern medicine and modern sanitation, couples bore many children, and many of those children died before their own time of reproduction. In 1790, when the first U.S. Census was taken, the Total Fertility Rate was almost 8 children per woman, believed to be among the highest in the world at the time. Benjamin Franklin wrote how children swarmed across the countryside like "a wave of locusts." But infant and child mortality was also high. Walk through an

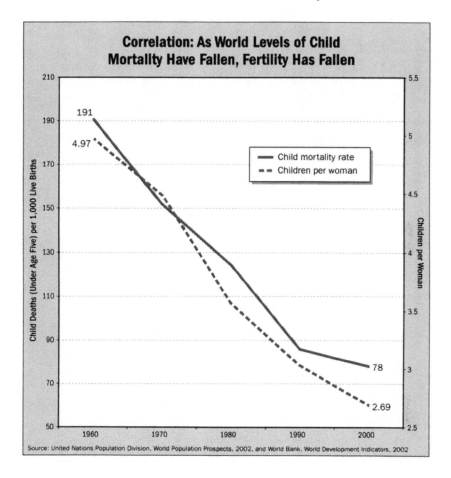

Correlation: As World Levels of Child Mortality Have Fallen, Fertility Has Fallen

Source: United Nations Population Division, World Population Prospects, 2002, and World Bank, World Development Indicators, 2002

old church cemetery one day and look at some of the tiny headstones. High fertility, high mortality. If many babies died, parents would have to conceive and bear many children in order to leave heirs and get help tilling the land. There was logic to that.

With changing medical conditions and improved public sanitation, infant mortality plunged. In 1900 in the United States, 165 of every 1,000 infants died before reaching their first birthday. Today the rate is 7. In Japan the infant mortality rate was 51 in the early 1950s, and 3 today. So, as Transition Theory has it, couples needed to conceive fewer children to replace themselves, and accordingly had fewer children. Low infant mortality yielded low fertility. With a very few temporary exceptions, high-high to low-low was the clear general trend in all the developed nations, with the low-low scheduled to settle in at about 2.1 children per woman.

But that's not what happened. Today, with the exception of just the minuscule Albania, every modern nation—44 of them—is below that 2.1 replacement level, almost all of them well below it. The only serious outlier is America, which according to the National Center for Health Statistics recorded 2.01 in the year 2002, just a bit below the replacement level. (Albania, total population 3.1 million, roughly the population of metropolitan Cleveland, isn't a very modern place anyway. Albania's fertility rate, now officially at 2.3, has fallen from 6.0 in the late 1950s and is probably now below replacement level.)

What happened to the equilibrated harmony of the Transition Theory? It ran into one problem: while most families with demographers in them have children, most children are not born to families with demographers in them. Young people make individual and private decisions about family size, often in the privacy of their bedroom. They are not concerned with distant population projections. They do not worry about the replacement rate. They do not care if the graceful curved line on the graph settles at 2.1 or below or above. For now, they don't seem to care much whether their own nation will grow, or shrink rapidly. In political science and sociology such mass personal behavior is often colorfully described as "people voting with their feet"—in other words, people move from farm to city, or from Mexico to America, based on individual personal decisions. But in the realm of demography that is only partially so: there has not been less sex, just less procreation.*

Acting without permission of the demographers, the peoples of Europe and Japan, and some American subgroups, began having fewer and fewer children. Individually, case by case, they created a collective revolution of falling propagations. In the late 1950s the European TFR was 2.7. In the early 1970s the rate was 2.16. Then, from 1985 to 1990, the number of children per woman in the developed world fell to 1.8 children per woman.

Now, the world had seen low fertility rates before, even below-replacement-level fertility rates. But such rates had occurred in times

---

*A survey conducted in 2001 by the condom maker Durex showed the Japanese with the lowest rate of sexual activity among 28 nations: 36 times per year. In first place was the United States with 124 times per year.

of plague, war, economic depression, famine, or great social disruption. Afterward, fertility rebounded. But, uniquely, in the modern nations during the 1980s this was happening without catastrophic factors, in a time of peace for these nations, albeit in the context of a generally quiescent cold war. (And when the cold war ended, fertility dropped even faster.) The modern economies were largely prosperous, in fact reaching a point of prosperity unmatched in human history, certainly so in the non-Communist part of Europe. Yet the 1.8 TFR was the lowest noncatastrophic such number ever recorded.

Moreover, most all signs pointed downward. So many factors were in the saddle that had historically tended to signal lower fertility. Scores of millions of people were moving from farms to cities; women were getting more education; contraception had become easily available; abortion had been legalized; feminism was coming on with a rush; women were more likely to be at work.

Another fifteen years went by. By 2000 the fertility rate in the modern countries had declined from 1.8 to 1.6 children per woman—24 percent below the replacement level. This figure included the United States, with 285 million people. But in the late 1990s the U.S. had a TFR of 2.0, higher by far than the 1.60 for the aggregate of all the More Developed Countries. To be sure, the American rate was below replacement, just as it had been for thirty years, but not much below, and bolstered by ongoing robust immigration. The European rate, however, was down to 1.42 in the 1995–2000 time frame.

There was one more turn of the ratchet yet to come. In the current time frame (2000–2005) the projected European TFR is estimated at 1.38 children per woman. That number is 34 percent below the replacement level. Japanese rates are almost identical.*

(The UN Population Division has some astonishing numbers on the percentage of women who have no children at the end of their childbearing years. These include: Germany 26 percent, Finland 21 percent, United Kingdom 21 percent, Netherlands 19 percent, Italy 19 percent, Luxembourg 18 percent, Switzerland 16 percent, Sweden 15 percent, Canada 14 percent, and Denmark 10 percent. The rate

*Sixteen European nations have rates at or below 1.3, including Spain (1.15), the Czech Republic (1.16), Hungary (1.20), Poland (1.26), Austria (1.28), Romania (1.32) and Germany (1.35).

for the United States, according to the National Center for Health Statistics, was 16 percent in 2002, up from 11 percent in the early 1970s. In 2003, Gallup asked American respondents over age forty-one who do not have children, whether they would not have children "if you had to do it over again." Only 24 percent said they would have "none," with the remainder specifying the number of children they wish they had borne.)

So beware of using the "More Developed" TFR, now 1.56, as a universal modern rate. I date myself, but the situation would be akin to reporting scores of the championship teams of the Chicago Bulls. One could write that Michael Jordan and Scotty Pippen had averaged twenty points in a game against the Los Angeles Lakers, when in fact Michael had scored thirty and Scotty had scored ten.

The Europeans are in the basement of fertility; America lives on the ground floor of its split-level house. The United States is the exceptional country in the current demographic scene. That point will be recalled frequently in this book. Among the modern nations, it has been three full decades since fertility has fallen sharply below replacement. The UN "medium variant" projection—which I believe is structurally on the high side—shows European population declining from 728 million souls today to 632 million by 2050, and then heading down to even fewer people with ever greater speed. The demographer-economist Samuel Preston is the former president of the Population Association of America and a leading light in the demographic club. A few years ago he estimated that even if European fertility rates miraculously jumped back to replacement-level immediately, the continent would still lose 100 million people by the year 2060.

How many people will the modern countries lose in the years to come? Many.

Here is the appropriate place to use the "Constant-Fertility Variant" (C-FV), one of the four projections published in the UN's *World Population Prospects*. The C-FV projects population figures *as if there were no changes in the fertility rates now prevalent.*

As indicated, the modern countries (America excepted) have very low Total Fertility Rates today. The UN broke fresh ground when it announced a TFR of 1.85, below the 2.1 replacement level. But for nations with low TFRs, that does not mean a decrease in fertility, but

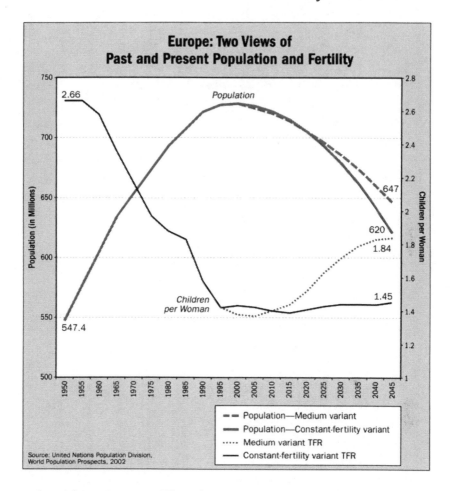

Europe: Two Views of Past and Present Population and Fertility

Source: United Nations Population Division, World Population Prospects, 2002

- – – Population—Medium variant
- — Population—Constant-fertility variant
- ····· Medium variant TFR
- — Constant-fertility variant TFR

rather a large *increase*. Thus the current German TFR is 1.35. Using the new level of 1.85 means going *up* by a half a child per woman, which is quite substantial. As we shall see, there is no evidence that such an increase is occurring. (The German Statistical Office uses a TFR of 1.4 children per woman in 2050 for its calculations.) There may even be signs that the trend is going the other way.

Consider Europe, the big fellow among the modern population groupings. Its population in 2000 was 728 million. Under the Medium Variant the European population falls to 632 million people in 2050. Under the (more appropriate) Constant-Fertility Variant the European population falls to 597 million people in 2050, an additional drop of 35 million people—a total shrinkage of 18 percent, and projected by the UN to continue falling. To do the arithmetic for you, this means 131 million fewer people in Europe. Joseph Chamie uses the C-FV frequently to explain what happens if nothing changes among low-fertility countries, and notes that despite massive efforts, no governmental programs have yet been able to raise fertility substantially.

Will such projections come to pass? As demographers emphasize, these are projections, not predictions. Overpopulation alarmists made their case by showing geometrically driven trends. Now New Demographers can use geometric progressions to show the impact of falling fertility. Demographers used to talk about the "doubling rate," the number of years it takes for a population to *rise* by 100 percent. These days one hears talk of the "halving rate," the number of years it takes for a population to *fall* by 50 percent.

But there is one difference. A population explosion notwithstanding, the world generally did quite well in the second half of the twentieth century, by most economic and social standards. We don't yet know whether that will prove to be the case as population falls. We don't know because the world has never seen anything like what is going on now. Should these rates not turn around fairly soon and fairly robustly, the ramifications are incalculable—or as the Italian demographer Antonio Golini mutters repetitively at demographic meetings, "Unsustainable, unsustainable."

What on earth is happening in these modern nations? One hears about many separate things, adding up to one big thing.

* The Japanese, it is said, are smack in the middle of a feminist revolution that lowers fertility. Some Japanese say a deeply troubled economy has added to the problem. In Japan, women who work and do not marry have been referred to by sociologist Masahiro Yamada as "parasite singles." The distinguished sociological journal *USA Today* quotes a forty-year-old Japanese single male this way: "Men don't want to spend time with their girlfriends, especially shopping." That's why birthrates are so low in Japan.

* In Italy it is said that Italian men now live in their familial homes into their thirties. Italian women will tell you, "They're mama's boys." That's why Italian fertility rates are so low.

* It is said that the Germans don't like children (*kinderfichlekeit*). That's why the German TFR is at 1.35. That's why the obstetrics wards are being converted to geriatric care.

* It is said that in Europe fertility is down because of double-digit unemployment in some places. Yes, that's why the European TFR rate is down to 1.38 children per woman in the 2000–2005 time frame, from 1.42 in the 1995–2000. (But fertility was also sinking when Europe was booming economically.)

* In Eastern Europe it is said that the economic dislocation due to the fall of communism must be considered. That's why the Eastern European rate is at 1.2 children per woman, only slightly above half the replacement rate.

* In Russia, there is a health crisis. That's why fertility is down (to an almost unbelievable 1.1) and why Russia is already losing population at the rate of about 800,000 people per year. (Before the fall of communism it was said that fertility rates were low because people had no hope in such grim and unfree societies.)

* And in Canada it sometimes is said that fertility is down to 1.5 because the French Canadians, who used to have bushels of children, now have few, having forgotten their alleged demographic plan ("The Revenge of the Cradle"—*la revanche des berceaux*) to take over the Dominion.

And so on, and so on, in all the modern, postmodern, industrialized, postindustrial, Information Age nations that make up what is called "Western Civilization" (except America). All these reasons appear to have some validity in greater or lesser degree.

But what is conveyed by the totality of these separate ideas? Why are these young Europeans and Japanese having so few children? It isn't war. They were born after the end of World War II. After almost half a century of vicious bloodshed among these very countries, there was a half-century of general peace, which not only continues but has made even the thought of one European country marching on another sound preposterous. This has been a great European achievement, made possible in large part by American military guarantees.

Can you imagine Germans marching into a faltering France? Germans can now get to the Eiffel Tower, without a visa, with just a fistful of Euros, and no need to accept a French surrender. After the Soviet Union engaged in self-dismemberment, the idea of Soviet troops pouring through the Fulda Gap and on into Western Europe became absurd. For now and the foreseeable future, the Russians aren't

marching anywhere into Europe. Their only march, one hopes, is toward democracy, civil order, an operative market economy, and better
health. (We shall have to wait a while to see how that turns out.)

Europeans are not having few children because of bad economic
times. These young Europeans grew up in a time of prosperity. For
example, real per capita income in the principally European countries
of the Organization for Economic Cooperation and Development
(OECD) was $9,977 in 1960 and $29,844 in the year 2000. The
numbers are in constant 1995 dollars. Incomes in the former Communist empire have been much harder to measure, but in those countries too, real income has climbed.

Greater income, especially discretionary income, yields interesting fertility dynamics. I visited Hungary in 1965 because Hungary
had a very low fertility rate and a particularly high rate of legalized
abortion. I asked the sociologist Rudolph Andorka what was going
on. He speculated that it was "*Kichi vad kochi*," a play on words in
Hungarian meaning "Child or car." (Hungarian spelling: "Kicsi
vagy kocsi.")

Within grim Communist parameters, Hungary was doing pretty
well economically. Not well enough, said Andorka, so that upscale
couples could afford to bear and raise a second child *and* own a car,
but often well enough to do one or the other. Many chose a car. Except for certain kinds of group travel, the cold war had made travel
outside the Communist bloc nearly impossible. A Hungarian could
no more hop into his own car and drive to nearby northern Italy for
a week's vacation than he could board a spaceship to the moon. But
if communism restricted travel and yielded low incomes, the system
did provide for vacations. (Some said vacations were easy to grant because the workers did so little on the job in the Communist command
economies that they were scarcely missed.)

Hungary is a beautiful country of 35,000 square miles (slightly
larger than South Carolina's 31,000 square miles). Owning a private
car in Hungary meant that someone in Budapest could drive to work
during the week instead of strap-hanging on a crowded bus. It meant
that on a weekend he could drive sixty miles west to the near shore of
Lake Balaton for a Sunday trip. Professor Andorka and I took such a
trip through a lovely pastoral region. The Balaton itself is sixty miles

long, running east-west. A motor trip to the far side could be a week-end adventure. With appropriate visas—not hard to obtain within the Soviet bloc of satellite nations—a week's vacation in Communist-but-cosmopolitan Prague (250 miles away) or at the Black Sea beaches in Bulgaria was a distinct possibility.

America is a car-crazy country. But as nations around the world have become wealthier, it has become increasingly obvious that the desire for the liberating force of personal transportation is universal. The progression often goes from scooter, to bicycle, to motor scooter, to automobile. Japan went below the replacement rate at about the same time as Hungary did, and at about the time when the word "mycar" came into the Japanese language. The word connoted a personal possession, "my own car."

The "child versus car" dilemma was of course not unique to Hungary. Cars and children share at least one thing in common: they are expensive, particularly so in urban surroundings. In Europe today, the cost of highly taxed petrol runs to about four dollars per gallon.

And "child or car" is an apt expression for more than just cars. What does a family decide when the choice is an additional child—versus a televison, hi-fi, stereo, washing machine, phone, computer, TiVo, DVD player, i-Pod, online service, cell phone, a trip to a Caribbean island, or tuition to a private school—and the list goes on and on. These days, throughout the modern world, there are lots of goods and services to buy—all made easier if you keep your family small.

Thirty-seven years after my 1965 visit with Andorka, in 2002, I was at work with a film crew in Rome doing interviews for a PBS special called "The Grandchild Gap." Here are some excerpts:

GIORGIO BENVENUTO (chairman of the finance committee in Italy's Chamber of Deputies): "Something peculiar has happened in Italy in recent years. The number of pets, the number of cats and dogs kept in the homes, has drastically increased. Multi-national firms producing pet foods are booming in our country. Even if you turn on the television, you can't help but notice all the commercials for cat and dog food. This means that people miss having something to care for, to keep them company. Therefore I think that people realize this is a loneliness problem, that is, people feel lonely even in a crowd."

OLDER ITALIAN WOMAN #1: "On the whole, people tend to miss having grandchildren, just as one tends to suffer from not having had any children."

OLDER ITALIAN WOMAN #2: "Most of them tend to devote their life to animals."

OLDER ITALIAN WOMEN #1 AND #5: "It's true."

OLDER ITALIAN WOMAN #2: "Yes, they tend to turn their love toward animals . . . little dogs, cats."

OLDER ITALIAN WOMAN #5: "Dogs, cats."

OLDER ITALIAN WOMAN #1: "They are no substitute, however! Whatever people may say."

Later we filmed in Paris. The TFR was higher than in the land of the bottoming bambino, but the problem was still there. Some excerpts:

FRENCH STUDENT #1: "It's maybe financial problems. You got to pay for studies. . . . I think they prefer raising children in a good way and just have one or two instead of have three or more and not being able to pay for studies and what they really need."

FRENCH STUDENT #2: "The problem today is that if you want to wait until you have enough money to start a family, you end up too busy and you have no time for your children. And even if you decide you want to start a family right away, you probably don't have the money to support children, so you end up waiting anyway. In my opinion it's a vicious cycle."

BW: "Would you like to get married?"

FRENCH STUDENT #3: "Not now."

BW: "Not now. But someday?"

FRENCH STUDENT #4: "Yeah, in a long time. Perhaps."

FRENCH STUDENT #2: "Both my grandmother and my mother have always told me it was important to have my own career and my own savings and be able to assume my own financial responsibilities."

OLDER FRENCH WOMAN: "My son has a girlfriend, and his job, and his apartment, and I think he prefers that stability. I think it would be great if they had kids in a year or two, but for the moment that is not a priority for them."

OLDER FRENCH MAN: "The downside is that if you wait too long to have children, you are really too old by the time they have kids.

You're almost dead, in fact. You're too old to enjoy being a grand-parent. It's much better to have them earlier."

JEAN-CLAUDE CHESNAIS (senior fellow at the Institute for Demographic Studies in Paris): "We are living in a totally new world. . . . Nobody I know, no demographer, no social thinker could have imagined that societies could have come below, much below replacement fertility, and that so many couples would remain childless."

And so young Europeans had small families, and then smaller still. If things proceed as expected, this postwar Euro-Japanese generation will live longer lives, in healthier circumstances, than any previous cohort of humanity. By any historical collective standard, the postwar generation has it all, or almost all. It has made individual decisions with its own best interests in mind. It wanted cars and vacations abroad. Women wanted education and career choices. It wanted its children to be well cared for and to attend good schools. And it decided to have fewer children than any cohort in human history. Individually, it apparently made sense.

As a libertarian on many issues, I salute free people making free choices in free nations. But collectively, unless something changes, and changes fairly quickly, these modern nations will go through a stark depopulation or an unwanted and turbulent flood of immigration to fill needed jobs, particularly jobs needed to care for the great expected growth in the numbers of elderly. In Europe, unwanted immigrants have typically been North African Arabs, or Turks to Germany. After the tragedy of 9/11, already hostile attitudes toward Muslim immigrants have intensified.

In the abstract I doubt that most Italians, Spaniards, Germans, Frenchmen, Poles, Hungarians, Romanians, or Japanese seek a future world with their national population an ever-diminishing number, and a waning of their individual national identities (though some Europeans do note that theirs is a "crowded continent"). But it will not be easy to turn around the trend.

DOES RUSSIA BELONG in the company of Developed Countries? That's where it is in the UN statistical scheme of things.

I have two colleagues at the American Enterprise Institute who pay particular attention to Russia. Leon Aron is one. He came to the

United States from Moscow in 1978. Later he spent ten years writing the definitive and magisterial biography of Boris Yeltsin, published in 2000.

Leon travels periodically to Russia and is in regular communication with his sources there. He thinks, all things considered, that Russia is doing pretty well. He sees a Russia generally friendly to the West and to America, with democracy generally embedded, with 40 percent of its households connected to the internet, unilaterally disarming, with average income rising at 6 percent annually, with 70 percent of the GDP in private hands, with a flat tax of 13 percent on personal income that Vladimir Putin says is "the lowest in Europe," and with forty-two cars per hundred people in 2001 as compared to eighteen in 1990. According to Aron, the Russians are on their way. He is concerned about the apparently growing autocracy of the Putin regime, as well as scandals, political machinations, and health problems, but remains optimistic.

Nick Eberstadt also pays a lot of attention to Russia, but most of his investigations have to do with searching through books of international, national, and local data and trying to figure out what they might mean. Unlike me, Eberstadt is a real demographer. He holds a chair at the American Enterprise Institute and for more than twenty years was a visiting fellow at the Harvard University Center for Population and Developmental Studies.

Eberstadt sees Russia as a broken nation, a demographic basket case, losing population by nearly a million people each year, with a TFR of 1.14, one of the lowest in the world, slated to lose about 30 percent of its population by 2050 according to UN projections, and with an age-standardized death rate among men almost 40 percent higher today than in the 1960s, according to Moscow's official figures. (The female death rate is also up, but by much less.) For Russian men, life expectancy dropped by about four years during this time. Moreover, the high mortality rates are concentrated among men of working age (age 20–64), likely making future economic growth more difficult, according to Eberstadt.

The demographer Murray Feshbach of the Woodrow Wilson International Center for Scholars notes that 50 to 60 percent of Russian children suffer from a chronic illness. Abortion rates (used as a very common means of contraception in Russia) are very high, and approximately 10 to 20 percent of Russian women become infertile after abortions.

Beyond these figures is the HIV/AIDS situation. Estimates differ. As of 2002 the sero-positive population in Russia seems to be in the one to two million range, somewhat more than 1 percent of the population. (The rate of "excess deaths" from HIV/AIDS was about the same in Russia and in America in the 2000–2005 time frame, according to UNPD data.) About 300,000 hardened criminals are coming out of Russian prisons each year, many of them with either HIV/AIDS or drug-resistant tuberculosis. Thus there is fear that the rate may increase, and that Russian officials are not paying sufficient attention to the situation.

Considering these indicators, does Russia belong in the ranks of the More Developed Nations?

Are Leon's and Nick's views compatible? They may well be. Russia appears to be on its way up from a dank cellar. It is a riven society, with some young, upwardly mobile, urban individuals leaving the poor and sick far behind. Will it stay that way or turn more egalitarian as the years roll on? It is not polite to consider "trickle down" economics. After all, we've been told by generations of liberal politicians that trickle-down is feeding the sparrows by feeding the horses. But it often has worked. Russia today doesn't really deserve the "More Developed" label. But I'd guess that it will in 20 to 30 years. (Anyway, who's going to say "No" to a mere label for a nation like Russia, which in 2000 still had about 6,850 nuclear warheads, some of them still operational?)

SOLUTIONS? The forthcoming dramatic depopulation of Europe and Japan will cause many problems. Populations will age, the customer base will shrink, there will be labor shortages, the tax base will decline, pensions will be cut, retirement ages will increase. Some of these problems are major, some only seem major but over time may be dealt with more easily than expected.

But is there a silver bullet, one macro solution? In fact there may be at least two. The distinguished Australian demographer Jack Caldwell believes that in a few decades Europeans will wake up to what is happening, decide they want their nations to exist, and will start having more babies. That is surely possible, but it will be a slow haul. Typically the phenomenon has been viewed on the upside: fertility rates may sink below replacement, but populations can continue to grow for many decades because there is so much "breeding stock" from cohorts born twenty or so years earlier. Consider Brazil: its TFR is now just about at replacement, and falling, but from 2000 to 2050 its population is nonetheless projected to grow from 172 million to 233 million.

But the same momentum works on the downside. Europeans may follow Caldwell's scenario and decide twenty-five years from now that they should have more babies. But where will the requisite number of parents come from? Surely not from the hollowed-out shells of Dutch, Italian, German, Hungarian, and Greek cohorts born during the birth dearth, unless they decide to have, say, four or five children per woman, which certainly doesn't seem to be likely.

The second solution is simpler: immigration. The modern countries are generally rich, certainly compared with the poor countries of the world. Wouldn't poor people want to go to rich places?

Modern countries in a low fertility spiral will need workers. The headline news is of the sort that says Germany will give visas to some Indian computer experts. That's fine, but much of that kind of work can often be produced off-site in Hyderabad and Bangalore, and delivered by pressing the "Send" button. Such is not the case with other types of service workers, particularly at the lower end of the occupational spectrum. After all, who will take care of the burgeoning numbers of old people around the world? Who will empty the bedpans in nursing homes? Who will wash the dishes? Nannies can be an exception, sometimes marrying a millionaire; most are poor immigrants. Who will mow the lawns? Who will make up the rooms in hotels? It is not likely to be Germans born of German one-child families, and raised as "Little Kaisers." (In China they call the only child the "Little Emperor.") If such menial tasks are to be done, they will likely be done by immigrants or their descendants—in the German case, typically Turks. This is by no means a new pattern: immigrants start out at the worst jobs; their children and grandchildren do better. But will these nations with 10 percent unemployment rates welcome more immigrants? With open arms? Everything we know about the politics of Europe and Japan says "No."

A recent UN publication, "Replacement Migration" (2001), gave some estimates of needed immigration under certain scenarios. It caused a firestorm in Europe, to the point where the European Union issued a statement telling the UN Population Division to mind its own business.

Consider Europe according to "Replacement Migration": Today Europe has more than twice as many people as the United States, but the whole continent takes in a net of 376,000 immigrants per year, about a third of the American number. In order to keep a *total constant population*, that European immigration number would have to rise to 1,917,000 per year, an annual increase of more than *500 percent*. To maintain a *constant age group of workers age 15–64*, the number of immigrants would have to rise to 3,227,000 per year, an annual increase of more than *900 percent*. The UNPD also calculated what it would take to keep the *dependency ratio* constant, that is, the proportions of working-age persons to those over age 65 and under 15. That would require an annual immigration of 27,139,000, an increase of more than *7,100 percent*. That is not likely to happen.

These were big, tough numbers when they were published in March 2000. The majority of immigrants who come to Europe are Muslims, mostly Arabs. Even after decades of residence, most have not integrated into their host societies, or been allowed to. The immigrant assimilation ethic is not there. A Dutchman is born Dutch, talks Dutch, eats Dutch, and has Dutch ancestors. That is the pattern, though there are a few exceptions. Among the lower classes in Germany there is substantial intermarriage between Germans and the offspring of Turkish immigrants. Some Pakistanis came to England as an entitlement of their membership in the British Commonwealth and have experienced some social integration. A black immigrant from a former Commonwealth country may be regarded as "British."

But these are exceptions. Many of the immigrants in Europe do not vote. In many nations they and their offspring typically have great difficulty achieving citizenship. In Italy it takes about fifteen years for legal immigrants to become full-fledged citizens (unless they have an Italian ancestor). Most Europeans believe that the presence of Muslim immigration has increased crime, which is quite probably correct. As a recent French official report—never released—showed, the rise in anti-Semitism in Europe is in large measure fueled by Muslim immigrant populations (although Europeans needed no lessons in anti-Semitism).

And all that was the situation *before* 9/11. Since then a European-wide dragnet has been draped over Muslim residents who come from countries that have been involved in terror. Some European countries have called for the expulsion of Muslim immigrants, or have made it much harder for Muslim illegals to enter the European zone, or have cut back on the admittance of refugees.

So neither elementary solution to the declining birthrate will be easy. Even the solid rise in fertility that Jack Caldwell speculates about would take many decades to reverse the coming depopulation. And immigration is resisted and resented.

In early 2004, UN Secretary-General Kofi Annan issued a vigorous statement supporting more immigration to Europe and more humane treatment for its immigrants. But the secretary-general lacks standing in this situation: he is elected by countries, not by voters.

This is not a simple situation for the Europeans, nor for the Japanese. They find themselves in a demographic ditch of monumental proportions. A commercial question will be explored in a later chapter, but I ask it here as an appetizer: Is it attractive to invest in a company that does domestic business while the numbers of its domestic customers grows fewer and fewer?

The weirdness of the current situation may be seen, somewhat simplistically, in this way. For much of the first half of the twentieth century, the peoples of Europe and Japan slaughtered each other or their neighbors partly in order to pass along their seed ideologically and demographically. Then, during the second half of the century and now on into the twenty-first, a new attitude has appeared: "To hell with all that." They now hardly bother to have babies. This is not necessarily bad news; we shall speculate about that. But if someone understands it, please explain.

CHAPTER THREE

Less Developed,
Less Fertility

WE HAVE BECOME ACCUSTOMED to think of the Less Developed Countries (LDCs), alias the "Third World," as the place where the population explosion goes Bang! Images race across our minds: many small children trailing a weary mother living in rotten slums and favelas in sprawling, ever-growing, and unmanageable cities, drinking unsanitary water, under horrible health conditions, with a standard of living hardly worth the phrase. Or there is the rural model: even more children, even greater poverty, illiterate and broken men and women hopelessly trying to scratch a living out of tired land, often victims of diseases long since vanished from the modern world. Often, civil war rages.

There is enough truth to such a description to make grown men cry. There are also more hopeful aspects to the situation, particularly on the demographic side. Yet they seem to be rarely discussed.

As recently as 1965–1970 the TFR of the LDCs was 6.0 children per woman. By 1985–1990 the rate had fallen to 3.8—a very substantial drop, but a very high level. In the 2000–2005 time frame, the TFR in the LDCs is 2.9 children per woman, and actually somewhat lower because we are near the end of that period.

Such a demographic movement is the most rapid fertility free-fall ever. The cause? All the traditional ones—urbanization, education,

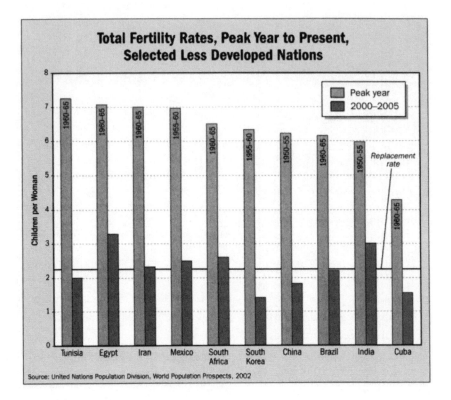

Total Fertility Rates, Peak Year to Present, Selected Less Developed Nations

Source: United Nations Population Division, World Population Prospects, 2002

women in the work force, contraception, abortion—and the intensification of a somewhat new one. The birth dearth has gained steam among *poor and uneducated women,* breaking some old rules. We shall explain later.

Which countries qualify as Less Developed? All those that were not originally categorized as More Developed—that is, the poor countries. But since that classification system took effect in the 1960s, some of the poor countries have become not-poor countries. Perhaps the most notable is South Korea. In 1960 the per capita income in South Korea was $1,325 per year (in constant 1995 U.S. dollars). In 2000 it was $13,199, moving toward European levels. Like the European nations, South Korea is a democracy. The UN's 2002 volume carried its TFR at 1.4 children per woman, a European level. But it is still counted as an LDC because it once was. Taiwan has a similar history, though it does not receive a separate page in the UN data volume because China says Taiwan is part of China. These days most of the 22 million residents of Taiwan apparently don't agree, but there's not much arguing with China, the world's largest country, with its 1.3 billion people and growing fleet of nuclear missiles.

Still, the LDC is not a bad classification. In broad strokes it is composed of all of Latin America, Africa, and Asia (with the Pacific exceptions of Japan, Australia, and New Zealand). These regions do indeed make up the poorer part of humanity, though there are substantial disparities among them.

The two most populous nations in the world, China and India, are LDCs. In the year 2000, China had 1.28 billion people and India 1.02 billion. They are the only two nations in the billionaire's club; no one else is even close. The United States was in third place with a mere 285 million people, about one-fourth that of China and one-third that of India. One of every three people in the world today is either Chinese or Indian. Each of the demographic billionaires have interesting demographic tales to tell.

IN THE LATE 1960S, China had a Total Fertility Rate of 6.06 children per woman, its peak year. That was almost exactly the average rate at the time for all the Less Developed Countries (6.01). Thirty years later the Chinese rate had fallen to 1.8, well below replacement.

What happened? In 1978 the Chinese government, then still led by Chairman Mao, instituted a "one child" policy: national family planning, with a coercive enforcement mechanism. Officially, no Chinese couple was permitted by the government to bear more than one child.

Enforcement required a top-down bureaucracy of massive proportions. In cities (where the rules were most stringently applied), block captains kept close tabs on every female in their designated area. How many children did the woman have? Was she pregnant? Had she missed her menstrual period? Because the Communist government had near-total control of the country, effective pressure could be brought to bear to bring fertility rates down rapidly. What kind of pressure? Loss of a woman's job, in a country where the government at that time was just about the only employer. Loss of her husband's job. Loss of a residence permit, in a country where the government owned just about all the housing. Sometimes there were forced sterilizations after the birth of a first child. If all else failed, a woman pregnant with a second child could be forced to abort the fetus. The coercive Chinese program worked, but not totally. The stated recent Chinese TFR is 1.8, far higher than the one-child family rule.*

Many human rights activists and some population activists regarded this policy as thoroughly evil, placing the state in total control of an intensely important and personal matter. That's my view. Some population activists thought that playing the China card in that way was an appropriate, if difficult, policy. China already had a population of 729 million people in 1965, with a growth rate of 2.6 percent a year—very high, a rate that would double the population in twenty-seven years. They accepted the Chinese government's view that the country would never realize economic growth unless population growth could be brought under control, quickly and forcibly.

Ultimately the matter became politicized. The United States refused to let any of its contributions to the UN Fund for Population Activities go to aid population control that included forced abortions. The UNFPA said that U.S. money wasn't going for that purpose, that funds were only helping China use other methods of family planning, and that coercion or forced abortion wasn't that common anyway.

One root of the debate concerned the question: Did population growth curtail economic growth? Another question emerged among geopolitically minded: If population ultimately plays an important role in creating power and influence, wasn't America better off if China—a potential adversary—had fewer people in the long run, no matter how repugnant their population policies were today?

---

*A commission has been appointed by the Chinese government to study the policy. Demographer Daniel Goodkind of the International Program Center of the U.S. Census Bureau estimates that the Chinese Total Fertility Rate is 1.65, below the UN's listed TFR of 1.83. Goodkind's data is based on official information from the Chinese National Bureau of Statistics, which probably means the UN 2004 data mid-century projections will come down. Thus the UN's TFR estimate is higher than that suggested by recent official data. According to the Population Reference Bureau, the rules have been implemented irregularly. Urban couples are typically limited to one child, but rural couples are allowed two children if the first is a daughter. What would happen if restrictions were lifted? If the TFR went up to, say, 2.0 children per woman, it would mean about 1.4 million additional births per year, and something like an additional 70 million people by 2050.

What happened in China after the one-child policy was put into effect? In successive five-year time blocks the TFR fell from 6.06 children per woman in 1960–1965 to 4.86 five years later, to 3.32, to 2.55, to 2.46, to below replacement at 1.92 in 1990–1995 and to 1.80 in 1995–2000. Both the 2000 and 2002 UN volumes showed the Chinese TFR at 1.8 children per woman. Obviously something very significant had happened. The Chinese TFR had dropped by 4.26 children per woman over the course of just forty years!

How to put that Chinese fertility decline in perspective? Not so easily. During the same time, in all the Less Developed Countries excluding China, fertility had declined from 6.16 children per woman to 3.3, that is, a drop of 2.8 children. That too was an enormous change, but less than the Chinese unfree-fall of 4.26.

On the other hand, just across the Yellow Sea from China another peasant society was also transforming itself. The South Korean TFR had been 6.33 in the late 1950s—and just 1.41 children per woman in 2000–2005. As mentioned, it was then re-reported by the government at 1.17 for 2003! Thus the South Korean TFR had dropped by 5.16 children from its peak year to the present, starting higher and falling faster than China's, to a lower point. The South Koreans did this without a coercive reproductive policy and with rapid economic growth up toward European levels.

A similar sort of story can be told about Taiwan. By 1999, according to the U.S. Bureau of the Census International Data Base, the Taiwanese TFR was 1.55 children per woman. (The 1998 rate was lower, 1.47 children per woman, believed to have been linked to the "Year of the Tiger," regarded as inauspicious for female births in Chinese societies.)

The below-replacement story was not just one of modern countries and a few exceptional LDCs. When the 2000 revisions were published, sixteen LDCs had fallen below the replacement level, just like China. When the 2002 revisions were published, twenty LDCs showed below-replacement rates, and the number was rising, with Brazil and Mexico expected to join this group soon.

Beyond the coercion needed to enforce it, there is another problem with the national ideal of a one-child family. Nick Eberstadt has written about life in such circumstances. Were such a world to come about, it would be one where children grew up without brothers or sisters, without uncles, aunts, or cousins and with as many as fourteen parents, grandparents, and great-grandparents (assuming rising life expectancies). In these nations the classic diagram of the "population pyramid" would soon look like a "population pole." In another words, in a one-child family, the child's only direct relatives are all ancestors.

Would that change the nature of our behavior? It might. For one example: Compared to parents with three children, parents with one child might not allow their child to take the reasonable risks associated with learning about the world. For another, while the data is not locked in, it is apparent that sex ratios in China are changing rapidly. Eberstadt reports that in China's 1953 and 1954 censuses there were 104–105 boy babies to 100 girl babies, about normal. In the 1982 census the ratio was 109. In 1990 it was 111, then 116 in 1995, and 118 in the November 2000 count.

Why? First a powerful cultural preference for sons. Second, sub-replacement fertility due to the one-child family rules. Third, the widespread availability of prenatal sex selection through sonograms and other technology, and subsequent abortion based on the sex of the fetus.* This can produce a major problem in the future. It is likely that in the decades to come 10 to 15 percent of Chinese men will be "unmarriageable" victims of a "bride shortage." In theory this would further lower Chinese fertility. Other potential examples of changed behavior are presented in Chapter Thirteen.

The Chinese situation is a prime example of the powerful role of "momentum" in modern demography. Consider carefully how it works; it is a crucial aspect of the New Demography.

Every birth, at the moment of delivery, requires both a woman and a baby. The baby's birth is reflected in current fertility rates. But what about the mother? She was not born today, nor born yesterday. She was born, let us say, about a quarter of a century ago, in 1975–1980. At that time the fertility rate in the Less Developed

---

*Unnatural sex ratios were also apparent in other Asian nations in the 1980s and 1990s, including Taiwan, Singapore, South Korea, and Hong Kong. Those ratios, but not China's, now seem to be reversing somewhat.

Countries was not the current 2.9; it was 4.6 children per woman. That means that there is a fat cohort of young potential mothers—today. Even if they bear relatively fewer children, even somewhat below the replacement rate, for a while population will still rise. That's how momentum works.

Thus China's fertility rate fell below replacement in the early 1990s, but its total population will grow until about 2025 before leveling off and shortly thereafter beginning a decline. And the growth until 2025 will be substantial. China's population in 2000 was 1.28 billion; in 2025 it will be 1.45 billion. That increase is a modest 13 percent, but it adds up to 170 million people—a massive increase, about equal to the current population of Brazil, the world's fifth-largest country.

Because of the momentum effect, one of the major arguments in population circles today is not so much *whether* the fertility averages for the less developed countries will fall to replacement levels and below, but *when* it will happen. If the decline to replacement level and below proceeds relatively quickly, the results from momentum will be relatively small. There will be fewer people of reproductive age twenty or thirty years from now, about when total global population might begin its decline. That would make it harder to reflate population numbers (if that is then considered desirable). And total global population numbers would be lower.

But if the decline in fertility happens more slowly, the momentum effect will push forward the time when global population begins to decline. Demographers who believe that current population growth is essentially harmful, like John Bongaarts of the Population Council, insist that we must act as quickly as possible to bring the LDC fertility rates down quickly, mostly through more extensive family planning and economic aid. (Remember, population will grow from about 6 billion to 8 billion before declining.)

In either case, at least according to the remarkable new UN medium variant projections, global population will be officially declining. Many of us saw this coming years ago; making it "official" is what makes it remarkable. Such a story, promulgated by the UN, headlined by the *New York Times*, couldn't be just a one-day story. It was a two-day story.

CONSIDER NOW INDIA, the only nation other than China whose population numbers go into ten figures—just over a billion in the year 2000. As recently as the early 1970s, Indian women were bearing an average of about five and a half children (5.43). Then fertility began plummeting, reaching 3.01 in the current estimate. Some of the large Indian provinces are already below replacement level. But the national TFR is still above replacement, and the Indian median age, at twenty-three, is lower than the Chinese median age of thirty. In large part because of momentum, intensified by a young age structure, India will be growing faster than China. Indeed, by about 2035 India is expected to overtake China and become the most populous nation in the world. Its population in 2045 is projected to break the 1.50 billion mark, still climbing to about 1.53 billion by 2050, by which time sparse China would have dwindled to a mere 1.40 billion people and India would soon begin its own population decline.

Like China, India has also tried to limit population growth, sometimes pushing close to the limits of coercion, occasionally crossing it. When Indira Gandhi was prime minister (1966–1977; 1980–1984), bonuses were given to women who had their tubes tied after a pregnancy. That is legitimate: a woman was encouraged to act in a certain way by a governmental carrot. For a man, a payment of a few rupees was tendered if he agreed to a vasectomy. Vasectomy peddlers received a bonus for each peasant male he could bring to the clinic for a vasectomy. Such is the way social engineering works.

But in 1975 Mrs. Gandhi declared Emergency Rule, the equivalent of martial law, undermining India's great claim to fame as the world's largest democracy. Encouraged by her son Sanjay, she applied pressure to meet sterilization quotas. Public employees' salaries were tied to the number of "acceptors" they brought in for sterilization. Fines and imprisonment were threatened. Food rations were withheld from the unsterilized. In some cases, procedures were performed without the woman's knowledge. That is not legitimate, it is clearly coercive.

(Some in the population business were pleased by the policies. Robert McNamara, then president of the World Bank, stopped off in India during the Emergency Rule and applauded "the political will and determination shown by the leadership at the highest level in intensifying the family planning drive with a rare courage of conviction."

And Paul Ehrlich was critical of the United States for not supporting *mandatory* sterilization of all Indian men with three or more children. He said, "We should have volunteered logistic support in the form of helicopters, vehicles, and surgical instruments. We should have sent doctors. . . . Coercion? Perhaps, but coercion in a good cause.")

Such coercive practices lasted only a few years. India is a democracy, and when voters got wind of what was going on, Mrs. Gandhi was voted out of office. The issue of coerced family planning was one of the reasons. Democracy offers people a powerful role in how they choose to run their lives. In general this is a blessing: how leaders think people ought to behave is not always the way people want to behave.

In India, particularly in the rural areas, boy babies are valued more than girl babies. And so today sex selection has become an issue. Technicians travel from village to village with portable sonogram instruments, telling pregnant women the sex of their fetus. This has apparently already led to abortion based on gender. The normal ratio of boys to girls at birth is 103–105 baby boys for every 100 baby girls. Today in India, according to its 2001 census, for every 100 girl babies born there are 108 boy babies born. The ratio may well climb still higher, as it has in China.

Beyond the billionaire nations, most of the rest of Asia is following apace. Asian fertility has fallen from 5.7 in the 1965–1970 period to 2.55 in the current period. Many of the smaller Asian nations are already well below the replacement level, including South Korea, Sri Lanka, Thailand, Taiwan, and Singapore. In addition, some of the former Soviet republics have also fallen below the 2.1 threshold, including Kazakhstan, Ukraine, Armenia, Azerbaijan, and Georgia.

MANY DEMOGRAPHIC RULES have been broken on the road to the New Demography. First was probably the one about Catholics. Because of the policy of the Catholic church regarding birth control and abortion, it was assumed that Catholic fertility worldwide would be higher than Protestant rates. For many years that was true. In the United States, for example, the Catholic TFR in the early part of the twentieth century is believed to have been substantially higher than the Protestant TFR. Italian immigrants, for example, were known for their large families. But that changed. These days the U.S. fertility rates for Catholics and Protestants are about the same. Attitudinal surveys also show that Catholics and Protestants have similar views on birth control and abortion.*

More dramatic than the American situation is what has happened in Europe. Through 1980–1985 the nations in Europe that were predominantly Catholic (mostly Southern European) had higher fertility rates than those European nations which were predominantly Protestant (mostly Northwestern). Thus in 1970–1975 the peoples in the nations of Southern Europe had a TFR of 2.54 children per woman while the Northern Europeans had already fallen below replacement level (2.08 children per woman).

Then, for no apparent reason, the bottom fell out of Southern European fertility. The current rate in Southern Europe is calculated at 1.32 children per woman, an amazingly low number. Among the lowest fertility rates in the European arena are the Italian (1.23) and the Spanish (1.15). Meanwhile, Northern European rates have also declined substantially, to 1.6 children per woman, but are higher than the Southerners after starting much lower. In Europe today, Protestants have more children than Catholics.

In the early 1960s the TFR for all of South America was 5.8 children per woman. Observers who worried about population growth looked at this essentially Catholic continent and shuddered. How could fertility ever be expected to fall quickly? South America would be overflowing with humanity.

It is not, and it will not be. Today the South American TFR is at 2.45 and falling quite rapidly. The sharp decline is led by the biggest Latin American country, Brazil, which had a TFR of 6.15 in the early 1960s. Today the listed Brazilian rate is 2.2, but Brazilian demographers say that the TFR has already crossed into below-replacement territory and that further declines are clearly in the off-

---

*In 1976 Earl Butz, the U.S. secretary of agriculture, said several things he shouldn't have to a reporter. One concerned the pope and contraception, and was delivered in a mock-Italian dialect. "He no play-a the game," said Butz to the reporter, "he no make-a dah rules." You may inscribe in your book of practical politics: Don't make jokes about the pope. Some Catholics were offended. Butz was fired. The birthrates did not change.

ing. What is more remarkable about the Brazilian situation is that there has never been a government program or policy to reduce fertility (though nongovernmental organizations in Brazil have vigorously promoted fertility guidance). That fact is not often stressed in the population-alarm industry.

The second-largest Latin American country is Mexico, also predominantly Catholic, and of particular interest to the United States. The Mexican TFR was 6.96 in the late 1950s. Seven children per woman! By 2000–2005 it was listed as 2.50. As mentioned, many Mexican demographers report that the Mexican TFR is now at about replacement level and falling. This stark decline may well change immigration flows into the United States.

Economic development is supposed to correlate with low fertility, isn't it? But Argentina, Chile, and Uruguay, the three most economically advanced and Western-oriented modern South American nations, have TFRs of 2.4, 2.35, and 2.30, respectively. Their TFRs have fallen more slowly than the South American average. Why? I don't know. And the experts don't know either.

IS DEMOGRAPHY DESTINY? The question is always with us and often surfaces with particular urgency at times of international tension. Such a view arises with particular potency during each Israeli-Palestinian crisis. Israel, we are told, is under the demographic gun as well as under fire from homicide bombers.

In the *New York Times* in 2002, columnist Nicholas Kristof noted that Palestinians bear twice the number of children per woman as do Israelis, therefore making the Israeli settlements in the West Bank "steadily less tenable." But Kristof was a beaming optimist compared to historian Paul Kennedy (who in the 1980s wrote that Japan would soon surpass America as the world's economic powerhouse). Writing for the Los Angeles Times Syndicate, Kennedy wrote that "hundreds of millions, literally hundreds of millions" of young Arabs and Muslims will be on the warpath as a "demographic boiling-over" yields "overpopulation, poverty and young male frustration . . . to carry out attacks against the West, and Israel in particular," which will "obliterate Israel or drive it to some desperate action." Kennedy wrote that he was "incredibly gloomy." Calm down, Paul.

The Israeli-Palestinian conflict has been brutal and tragic. As this is written, no two-state arrangement between the parties seems imminent. But let us try to lift some of the demographic darkness from Professor Kennedy's brow. It may well be that Israel should leave the settlements, as Kristof says. It may well be that Israel is in for very tough times ahead, as Kennedy says. Demographic trends will play some role, but there is somewhat less there than meets the eye.

Just as the "Catholic rule" was broken, so too is the Muslim rule breaking. Almost unnoticed in the general dialogue, fertility rates in Arab and Muslim countries have been falling very rapidly in recent decades. Indeed, it would be remarkable were they not; it's been happening everywhere else.

Consider North Africa as a bloc, nearly total Arab. Forty years ago the Total Fertility Rate was 7.1 children per woman. Today it is 3.2 and sinking like a stone. Egypt is the most populous North African country. Its TFR was 7.1 children per woman in 1960–1965. It is now 3.3. The UN Population Division reports Tunisia's current TFR at 2.0 children per woman, below replacement.

Go east. Syrian fertility has fallen from 7.6 children per woman to 3.3, and is sinking. From peak year to the present, here are some other Middle Eastern numbers: Jordan, 8.0 to 3.6 children per woman; Iraq, 7.2 to 4.8; Saudi Arabia, 7.3 to 4.5. These are still very high numbers, but, again, falling very rapidly.

Go farther east. At its peak Iran's TFR was 7.0 children per woman in the early 1960s. It is now officially at 2.3 and dropping rapidly, quite possibly below the replacement level as you read this.

Other big Muslim countries that have also seen major declines include Turkey, Bangladesh, and Indonesia. Only Pakistan among the major Muslim nations remains with a quite high current TFR, 5.08, but Pakistani fertility has fallen by a whole child from the 1985–1990 time frame. It looks like the demographic transition is slowly finding its way to Pakistan, as it has globally.

Joe Chamie is not surprised at this development. His Ph.D. dissertation in 1976 and his 1981 book *Religion and Fertility* quite clearly predicted just what has happened. Chamie makes a universalist case for demographic decline. People are people. Sooner or later, Catholics behave like Protestants, Muslims behave like Christians.

The big question is whether it will be sooner or later. As I read the data, the answer is sooner.

Which brings us back to the Israelis and Palestinians. It is an inordinately complex demographic situation which involves differential fertility rates among Jews, Christians, Druze, and Arabs as well as immigration, emigration, Israeli Arab citizens in Israel, and Israeli ultra-Orthodox Jews who encourage high fertility among their members and have huge families. The great mystery about this situation is that no one seems to know what percentage of the ultra-Orthodox Jews fall away from their rigid faith as they age. Israel is a swinging place—even during an Intifada—and the temptations of modernism are great.

The bottom line is that the demographic situation for the Jews of Israel is not nearly as bleak as it is sometimes portrayed. In 2002 the Jewish Israeli TFR was 2.6,* and has been hovering at about that figure since 1990. It has a TFR higher than that of any modern country, the only one seriously above the replacement level, and far higher than the rate for Jews in the rest of the world. Why? I think much of the high Jewish fertility in Israel concerns the fifty-year war that the Israelis have been engaged in since their independence in 1948. Many Israeli families have had a third child as an "insurance policy," fearing that one child may be lost in combat or terror. There is a certain paradox here: Arab warfare and terror creates more Israelis. (Of course, we have also heard just the converse: that Israeli repression creates more Palestinian babies, to reconquer Israel.)

What about the Palestinians? The UN issues data for "Occupied Palestinian Territory." On average, OPT women are bearing 5.6 children, a very high rate but down from an estimated 8.0 as recently as 1970 and 7.0 as recently as 1985. Palestinians in the OPT watch television and see modern life, just as most all the world now does. And the Palestinians are deciding to have somewhat smaller families.

Both populations have grown. The current population of Israel is 6 million, up from an estimated 1.3 million in 1950. OPT population today is 3.2 million, up from 1.0 million in 1950. By the year 2025 the population of Israel is projected at 8.6 million. There has been

---

*Source: Statistical Abstract of Israel. In Israel proper, the Muslim TFR in 2002 was 4.6, the Christian rate 2.3, and the Druze rate 2.8.

much talk that the terror inflicted on Israel during Intifada II, and a long recession caused by the violence, will drive Jews out of Israel.

The "Second Intifada" began in 2000. Still, in 2002, 34,000 migrants came to Israel. That was, however, down from the 50,000–75,000 range of immigration between 1995 and 2000. The OPT is projected at 6.9 million in 2025. In short, two countries of about 6 to 8 million people each, living side by side, in peace or in war, one quite modern, one hopefully modernizing.*

Another often unnoticed fact impacts the Middle East situation. The Arab nations are vast in size but small in population. Those clichés about "vast seas of sand" are partially true. Beyond Egypt's roughly 75 million, there isn't an Arab nation with more than 35 million people, that is, approximately the population of California. The total population of all the Arab nations combined is about 284 million, approximately the size of the United States.

Many factors go into the idea of power—armed might, economic wealth, culture, natural resources, allies, technology, an educated citizenry, spirit, and, always important, numbers. While numbers play a role there, I do not believe the Israel-Palestine situation is one that will be settled principally due to demographic projections.

TALK TO PEOPLE who still want to play the population card and they bring up sub-Saharan Africa. Indeed, the fertility rate in the area is 5.4 children per woman—down from 6.6 as recently as 1980–1985, but still very high.

But several factors must be understood. By any relative standard, sub-Saharan Africa has few people. Like its neighbor in northern Africa, sub-Saharan Africa has only one large country, Nigeria, with

---

*For the record, the U.S. Census Bureau reported in December 2003 that the Arab ancestry population in America rose to 1.2 million during the 1990s, up from 860,000 in 1990 and 610,000 in 1980. The Census Bureau does not take data by religion, but independent studies show the Jewish-American population in the 5 to 6 million range. The total Muslim population is now estimated in the range of 1.9 million to 2.8 million. The study was conducted by the survey researcher Tom Smith of the University of Chicago and was commissioned by the American Jewish Committee. Some Muslim groups maintain that an earlier estimate of 6 to 7 million remains correct.

a population of 130 million people projected for 2005. In second place is Ethiopia with 74 million people projected for 2005. The Congo has 56 million people. South Africa has 45 million people. After that are a couple of countries roughly the size of California (Sudan and Tanzania) and a host of smaller countries that make up the 50 nations in the sub-Sahara. The total population of sub-Saharan Africa in 2000 was 653 million. In the year 2005 the total of all 50 nations of sub-Saharan Africa will be 733 million people, somewhat more than two Americas.

For a number of years the nation of Kenya was always held out as the basket-case example that proved the rule: the population explosion wasn't even close to running its course in some places. Indeed, as recently as 1980, Kenyan women bore an average of 7.9 babies and had stayed at about that level for some twenty-five years. It was a good example of ongoing, apparently intractable levels of high fertility, but in a global sense it didn't add up to a hill of Kenyans. The total population of Kenya in 1980 was only 16.4 million, less than that of Greater New York City. In 2005 its population is 33 million, but these days Kenya is barely mentioned in population dialogue. Its TFR, according to the UN, has fallen to 4.0 children per woman. In the 2005–2010 time frame, the TFR in Kenya is projected at 3.47, well below the U.S. rate (3.8) at the peak of the American Baby Boom in the late 1950s.

It has been said that Africa is the continent progress missed. That was misleading. It started out way behind in the race to development. But in some places, income has been moving up smartly. A number of sub-Saharan nations have moved to democratic governance, something that could not be said for the North African Arab countries. There has been ugly and gruesome warfare, some of it ongoing, but, alas, that is not so unusual in global history.

And then came the unexpected: a pandemic of HIV/AIDS, which frightened the world and ravaged whole regions of Africa. In 2000, UN demographers categorized 45 nations as "highly affected" by HIV/AIDS. Of those 45 nations, 35 were in Africa. Of 17.8 million "excess deaths" from HIV/AIDS projected from 2010 to 2015, 14.4 million will come from Africa. In Botswana, one of the African nations that has been doing rather well economically and is under democratic governance, about one of every three adults is HIV-positive. Botswana has begun a national campaign against the disease, automatically testing anyone who enters a hospital, and increasing the use of anti-retroviral drugs, with some apparent early success. Botswana is a tiny country (1.8 million), but South Africa is not (45 million people). The epidemic began its terrifying toll later in South Africa than in some other African nations, but by 1999 one of every seven adults in South Africa was estimated to be sero-positive. Seven countries in Africa have HIV rates at or above 20 percent.

So powerful is the demographic impact of the pandemic that UN demographers have concluded that South African life expectancy will fall from sixty-two to forty-seven years, while total population will actually decline from 2010 to 2025 before resuming slow growth. The 2002 edition of *World Population Prospects* officially "confirms yet again the devastating toll AIDS has in terms of morbidity, mortality and population loss." The number of highly affected nations has climbed from forty-five to fifty-three.

From 2000 to 2050 the UN projects that global population will be 479 million fewer than it would have been had AIDS not appeared and run to pandemic proportions. That is an astonishing number. The potential good news is that the UN projects that the probability of being infected by HIV/AIDS will decline significantly in the future, particularly after 2010.

While Africans have suffered most tragically from the epidemic, in other countries the ultimate impact may prove to be enormous. India, for example, is one of the fifty-three nations that are "highly affected." The rate of sero-positive persons in India is 0.72 percent, which is well below the 2 percent U.N. threshold for "highly affected." But because it is on a huge base of more than one billion people, it is included. Recent reports indicate that HIV/AIDS prevalence is growing in China, also a billionaire nation.

From the demographic point of view, there is an interesting side-light to the HIV/AIDS situation. The UNPD routinely includes data about what might be called an "epidemic of life," that is, the longer life expectancies that people around the world have become accustomed to, growing from forty-seven years at birth in 1950, to sixty-five years in the first years of the twenty-first century, to an estimated age seventy-four in the year 2050.

The AIDS data represents an "epidemic of death," and that too is blended into the UN forecasts. What is not in the forecast, however, is what we don't know. Are there are other epidemics to come? Is SARS (Severe Acute Respiratory Syndrome) a flash-in-the-pan epidemic or another dreadful plague waiting in the wings? What about avian flu? (The "Spanish Flu" epidemic of 1918 killed somewhere between twenty million and forty million people.) Will there be major wars? Will we see a great natural catastrophe? Will a terrorist strike make the three thousand deaths of 9/11 look small? (The three thousand deaths in a day in America was on a statistical base of 2.4 million deaths per year in America.) These sorts of unforeseeable factors can pull down a longevity forecast by a lot more than a year or two.

In America, for example, when the Congressional Budget Office makes its ten-year budget projection, it purposefully lowers growth rates somewhat to account for the possibility of a recession. The UN Population Division does not factor in potential catastrophes for even its longest-range projections. Obviously, were we to have such an occurrence again, population would sink even faster than outlined here.

PERIODICALLY the headline writers at the *New York Times* get things right. Recall, they did so on March 10, 2002, when they reported on the results of the UN proposal on population growth this way: "Population Estimates Fall as Poor Women Assert Control," with a subhead reading: "In India, Brazil, Egypt and Mexico, a Dip in Birthrates Defies Old Theories." A brief excerpt from this story, written by Barbara Crossette, is worth quoting:

> The decline in birthrates in nations where poverty and illiteracy are still widespread defies almost all conventional wisdom. Planners once argued—and some still do—that falling birthrates can only follow improved living standards and more educational opportunities, not outrun them. It now seems that women are not waiting for that day.

Indeed they are not, nor are their menfolk, who typically play a role in the child-creating process. Consider as a case in point what

has happened in Vietnam, a nation whose recent history is inextrica-
bly and tragically linked with that of the United States. As the Vietnam War raged in the late 1960s, the Total Fertility Rate in all of
Vietnam was 7.25 children per woman, and probably higher in the
North than in the South. It was an article of faith among the arm-
chair generals of the anti-war campaign that an American "body
count" campaign could never win because the North Vietnamese
were producing so much potential cannon fodder. Perhaps so.

America pulled out of South Vietnam. Less than three years later
the North Vietnamese army overran South Vietnam. It was not a
pretty picture. Tens of thousands of South Vietnamese fled the country, often as "boat people" risking perilous seas. Other South Vietnamese were killed or sent off to "reeducation camps." Many
Vietcong, the ostensible allies of the North Vietnamese, were also
treated harshly. Several of the fabled (and mocked) "falling domi-
noes" did indeed fall to Communist governments, in Laos and in
Cambodia, where a monumental genocide killed at least one million
Cambodians.

The Communist government of North Vietnam had all its ducks
in a row. The march toward socialist principles could commence in
earnest. A march did ensue—backward. The unified and independent
Communist nation of Vietnam suffered terrible economic conditions
for several decades. Not until the early 1990s when Vietnam, following China's lead, began adopting "communism with a capitalist face,"
or vice versa, did the economy begin to show vigorous signs of life.

But fertility sank rapidly before the economy improved. From the
high of 7.3 women in 1965–1970, it dropped to 4.02 twenty years
later. The 2000–2005 rate is recorded as 2.3, which is just about replacement level for an LDC like Vietnam, whose infant mortality rate
has fallen substantially but is still five times higher than that of modern nations. In short, Vietnamese men and women dramatically reduced their childbearing proclivities *before* economic advance.

So here is the state of play about fertility and economic growth:
In Less Developed Countries, when economic growth is percolating,
fertility falls; and when economic growth is sluggish, fertility also
goes down. The shorter way to say that is that in Less Developed
Countries, fertility is going down, way down.

A CRITICAL PART of the New Demography concerns what is called the "demographic bonus." Contrary to earlier ideas about economic growth in Third World economies, this one bodes well for the poorer nations.

The old argument was often presented in elemental terms. Population increases came from two basic sources: more old people living longer lives, and more babies coming into the world. Few of the elderly and none of the infants are in the productive work force. As these two groups rise relative to the working-age population, the per capita Gross Domestic Product either declines (as the pie gets cut into smaller slices) or does not rise as rapidly as it would have. Elaborate tables demonstrated that a sharp increase in population would create major demands for more schools, health care, housing, and most everything else. How could these demands possibly be met? The population alarmists said that the quickest and surest way to boost a Third World economy would be to reduce births.

But this view often left out one fairly obvious piece of the economic puzzle: babies become producers. Suppose in the mythical LDC nation of Ruritania, one million children per year are born. Five years later there would be five million children under the age of five, minus those infants and children who die before their fifth birthday. Because these children are economically inactive (so went the explosionist argument), the per capita GDP would be diminished.

But, first, modernization brought greater productivity. Notwithstanding the appalling level of poverty in most Less Developed Countries, the *rate* of per capita income growth in many LDCs has increased rapidly in recent decades, albeit often from a pathetically low level. On a relative scale, LDC per capita income growth has actually climbed faster than in the more developed nations, as we shall see later.

And, second, fifteen to twenty years after the birth of those mythical five million babies, they aren't babies anymore. They are potential young workers. They can work, and most of them do, despite high unemployment rates. They add to the GDP, and more than is generally assumed because so many are workers laboring in the "unofficial GNP," often working "underground" or "off the books." Many pay taxes. A famous Indian demographer noted that "every baby is born with a mouth and hands." A baby not only consumes when young but produces later on.

Meanwhile, as we have seen, LDC fertility has dropped substantially. Instead of five million babies and children under age five in Ruritania, there are now only, say, three million such infants and children. The "dependency ratio" has improved; there are fewer unproductive children drawing down family and governmental expenditures. The demographic bonus has arrived. And this process will continue as long as fertility continues to fall. This is exactly what is happening in the LDCs. Fertility has indeed fallen sharply, and all projections indicate that it will continue to fall. Accordingly, production should rise.

The familiar rhetorical rebuttal to this view is often as simple as it is wrong. Some ask: "But where will all the jobs come from? How can we create the jobs?" The answer is: There is no "we." Most of the jobs are "created" by "them," the people and the entrepreneurs, local or from outside the nation, not by "we" the governments, the economists, the planners. Adults need housing and food. The people in the LDCs want television and a bicycle, if not a motor scooter or a car. They work to gain that for themselves and their families, and they do so unless rigid governmental economic policies and corruption strangle economic growth—unfortunately an all too familiar story in the past, but getting better. As parents have fewer children, they can provide better education for those children. The next generation is more literate and more productive.

To a point, a fall in fertility can engender a virtuous cycle. If economic progress in per capita income is the sole variable, a family with two or three children will do better than a family with five or six children. An income of $100 each month in a family unit of seven (five children) yields about $14 per capita. The $100 in a family unit of five (three children) yields $20 in per capita income, almost a 50 percent increase.

But a simple decrease in fertility is not a panacea and never was. There are too many examples of nations that have fared very well with very high fertility rates. The nation with the largest population explosion in history has been the United States, growing from 4 million to nearly 300 million in 210 years while becoming the world's most prosperous nation.

The question before the house today is: Can a virtuous cycle turn into a vicious cycle in the LDCs? There is a commercial answer and an apocalyptic answer. One big part of the commercial answer is that things grow dicey when the fat cohorts of the Baby Boom age. Among the modern nations, that happens when Boomer babies born after World War II reach retirement age and there are few worker bees to pay into the pay-as-you-go retirement systems. That process is just beginning in those modern countries with relatively early ages of retirement. Sixty years from the end of World War II in 1945 puts us at 2005—now. Among the Less Developed Countries, this will happen decades later, because the decline in fertility began later and their populations will reach retirement ages later. But it will happen.

CHAPTER FOUR

America the Exceptional: The Baby Makers

THERE ARE More Developed Countries. There are Less Developed Countries. And there is the United States. Demographically, as in so many other ways, America is different.

The rich countries have very low fertility rates and populations that will shrink. The poor countries have sharply falling fertility rates, and populations that will grow for a while, but more slowly than expected. America fits into neither category. America is a rich country, the only one that is growing and has a fertility rate that is almost at the replacement level.

America continues to grow robustly for two reasons: apparently we have not lost the knack of having babies, and we still welcome a reasonable number of foreigners to our shores as residents.

Officially the United States is a statistical subset of the UN's category of "More Developed Regions." But America's differences from the "Rest of the West" are major. Perhaps the United States deserves a UN designation all its own, just as China has one. (The *World Population Prospects* volumes have a special category of data for "Less Developed Regions, Excluding China".) If the UN were to publish easily accessible data of "More Developed Regions, Excluding the United States," the remarkable story of modern American demographics would be seen much more clearly.

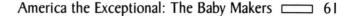

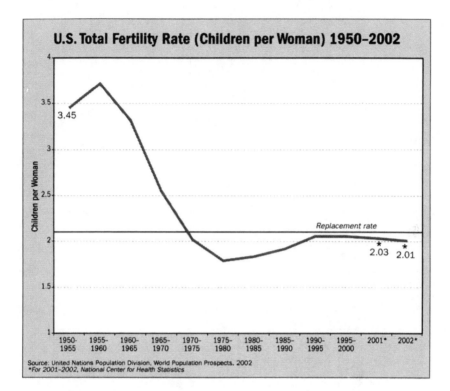

U.S. Total Fertility Rate (Children per Woman) 1950–2002

Source: United Nations Population Division, World Population Prospects. 2002
*For 2001–2002, National Center for Health Statistics

How is America different? Let us count the ways.

Big. America is the only significantly populous country in the West. The UN in 2000 showed America with 285 million people. By 2005 the American population should be about 300 million, growing moderately but solidly. To that can be added a few million more, in part because America is one of the few nations without a national identity and registration procedure, typically yielding an "undercount" in Census data (although the Census Bureau has been improving its enumeration procedures).

The next-largest truly modern country is Japan. It had a population of 127 million people in 2000–2005, well below Russia's 145 million and somewhat less than half the American number. Russia is already losing population; Japan will follow shortly. Both nations have steeply aging populations. By midcentury, remember, America will grow to about 400 million people, to about four times the number than expected in Japan, and aging more slowly.

In the year 2000 the population of all of Europe, stretching from Ireland to Siberia, including 47 nations, was 728 million people. By 2050, according to the UN Medium Variant projection, European population is estimated to be 632 million, a drop of 96 million people, and falling rapidly. (And perhaps significantly fewer, as we have seen and shall see again; the Medium Variant may not be the right way to look at Europe.) In short, Europe down 100 million, America up 100 million.

The farther out one goes, the more stark are the differences. Unless we know something will change—of which there is no evidence yet—it is not hard to get to a time when the United States will be more populous than Europe.

Now, granted, many things can change, and probably will. As Herbert Stein, my late colleague at the American Enterprise Institute, wrote, "A trend that can't continue, won't." It's not likely that Europe will fall to zero people at a certain date. On the other hand, in the world of demographics remarkable occurrences do happen—for example that seventy-five-fold increase in the U.S. population over the course of about two hundred years.

Fecund to none. Of the serious nations of the developed world, America has the highest TFR, about two children per woman, almost the replacement rate. We shall see if this will last.

What happened? For a while it seemed as if America would follow the European track of hyper-low fertility. In 1976, the year of America's Bicentennial, the TFR in the United States was 1.7 children per woman (in an economically unhappy time). How low was that? For the record, that number was below the then-current rate of France (1.9) and Japan (1.8). The all-Europe rate was 2.0. America, along with its modern counterpart nations, seemed to be heading into the same demographic ditch.

In the roughly quarter-century since then, Total Fertility Rates of most all the other modern nations have indeed fallen further. These included the settler nations of Canada and Australia, probably the two most similar to the United States in demographic structure.

But the TFR in America didn't stay down, it went up. Why? This would be an interesting demographic speculation for any nation behaving in such a quirky way. When it happens to the sole superpower, never more influential than now, it should become important news.

The United States in 1975–1980 was in the midst of what was then thought of as an economic implausibility: "stagflation." The Gross National Product was erratic, with two recessions, yet inflation soared. Could America's drop to 1976's TFR of 1.7 have been a reflection of the economic troubles? It would seem so. What could be worse for a young couple than high interest rates on a mortgage, high costs for goods and services while the real value of wages diminishes under the crush of inflation? With odd-even days of gas lines for fuel at high prices? Is that a propitious time to bear a first child? Is it a smart time to bear a second child?

So that's probably part of the answer. But how much a part? American fertility peaked in 1957 when Baby Boomers were being born at a TFR of 3.8 children per woman. The TFR then declined steadily: to 3.65 in 1960, to 2.9 in 1965, to 2.5 in 1970, and to 2.01 (just below replacement) in 1972. These were generally healthy economic times, yet the TFR was reduced by almost half. And rates were coming down in most all the modern nations regardless of how their respective economies were faring.

Why? For many reasons we will discuss later, including feminism, the education of women, women working, contraception, abortion, and urbanization.

What is more interesting is what happened after 1976. Slowly, very slowly in the beginning, American fertility began to rise. By 1980 the rate was 1.84, an increase of one-tenth of a child per woman from the 1.74 of 1976. By 1985 it was still 1.84, still in the European range. But from the latter part of the 1980s through the early part of the 1990s, as European fertility fell from 1.83 to 1.58, America diverged. Its rate in the latter 1980s climbed to 1.92, and then, in the first part of the 1990s, rose to the vicinity of 2.05, then dipped a bit just below 2.0, then climbed and dipped a bit again to the high 1.9s. In 2002 it was 2.01. The lesson here is: Do not count your chickens or children before they hatch. During this time Europe skidded to a stunningly low level of 1.4 children per woman.

Did something special happen in America in the late 1980s to kick off the American Baby Boomlet? Stagflation ended. It would surely seem that almost twenty years of unparalleled economic growth— roughly 1980 to 2000—in America played a role. After the short and steep recession of 1981–1982, America turned over a new page of economic history. Twenty years went by without anything resembling a deep or long recession. In 1992 the slogan posted in the campaign "war room" of Governor Bill Clinton of Arkansas read "It's the economy, stupid." On the stump, Clinton maintained that America was living through "the greatest recession since the Great Depression." But the final tally by the Bureau of Labor Statistics was that the recession of the early 1990s lasted only eight months, and economic growth fell by only 1.97 percent, not a terribly steep drop. In fact, by the time of the 1992 election the economy had been growing steadily for more than a year.

It would be simple enough to say that good economic times boost fertility. Parents have more money to raise children. But that is far less than a plenary answer. Over the decades, and centuries, greater income has been associated with falling, not rising, fertility. Recently, for example, Ireland has experienced a major economic boom, and its TFR has dropped from 3.8 children per woman in 1970–1975 to 1.9 in 2000–2005.

But America has some other unique features that would seem to be plausible candidates for a floor under fertility. Back in the year 1900, the rate of home ownership in the United States was 37 percent. The rate grew to about 45 percent by 1930, and then fell back to about 40 percent during the Great Depression of the 1930s and the outbreak of World War II. The end of the war and the subsequent growth of suburbia boosted the home-ownership rate. By 1960 it was about 60 percent. Another ascent began during the ongoing economically hot years of the 1990s, when low interest rates and more accessible mortgage loans pushed the ownership rate in 1999 to 67 percent.

By the year 2000 slightly more than half of all Americans lived in the suburbs, surely unique in the world. Almost two-thirds of all Americans had mortgage debt, also unique in the world. Home mortgages are often available for 80 or 90 percent of the cost of the dwelling, sometimes even more, a practice unheard of in most any other place in the world. The United States is probably the only nation in the modern world in which a majority of the population lives in single-family detached housing owned by the resident. Beyond that is the relatively low cost of gasoline: about two dollars per gallon in America versus about four dollars in Europe. That helps make it possible for people of ordinary means to own a vehicle big enough to

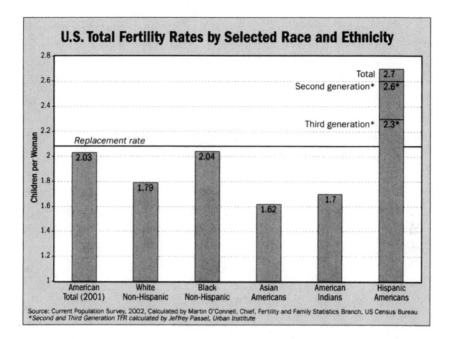

U.S. Total Fertility Rates by Selected Race and Ethnicity

Source: Current Population Survey, 2002, Calculated by Martin O'Connell, Chief, Fertility and Family Statistics Branch, US Census Bureau
*Second and Third Generation TFR calculated by Jeffrey Passel, Urban Institute

hold three children. (High gasoline taxes tend to be seen as regressive, even if coupled with tax rebates keyed to income. Well-to-do people can easily pay the extra money, but it may ration the amount of driving for a lower-middle-class person, or prevent that person from owning a second car.)

(In 2003 President Bush signed the American Dream Downpayment Act, designed for families that can afford mortgage payments but not the down payments on a first home. The legislation offers about $5,000 to low-income families buying their first home.)

And all that, of course, makes it easier to have children if you want to have children. Suburban homes typically have yards into which children can be tossed, and even small homes are expandable with dormers and add-ons and new wings. In Europe most people live in apartments. Some people own, some people rent. But three growing children in an apartment can often resemble a zoo or a madhouse. (Not that things are so calm in a suburban house.)

As I see it, it's good that America has had close to a 2.1 Total Fertility Rate, up from the Birth Dearth 1.7–1.8 pits of the mid-1970s. It's good that Americans face less of an "aging crisis" than other modern nations. There are, however, some caveats.

Again: it may not last. The TFR figure of 2.03 was recorded during the year 2001, mostly reflecting pregnancies from 2000, the year in which the Dow Jones industrial average peaked at 11,908. After the dot.com bubble burst, the 2002 TFR dropped a minuscule amount, to 2.01. My sense is that if America were to confront a 1970s-style stagflation, or any other sort of great difficulty, the TFR might drop back to that of the higher-level European countries. But because of ongoing immigration, it probably will not make much difference in population growth.

By 2001 America had completed the best twenty years of real economic growth in its history. Your author is an optimist but not a damn fool. The next twenty years may match the last twenty; I hope so, but we don't know.

There are some interesting sidebars from the latest data. In 1965, black fertility in America was 1.0 children per woman higher than that of whites (3.8 versus 2.8). By the early 1980s it was .4 children higher. Today the differential between non-Hispanic blacks and whites is about .2 of a child (2.04 versus 1.82). A principal cause for the closing of the gap was a sharp decline in teen-age fertility among blacks during the 1990s and early 2000s. From the early 1990s through today, the rate has fallen by almost half!

Asian Americans (1.8) and American Indians (1.7) have TFRs slightly below the all-American rates. The outlier rate is for Hispanic Americans at a TFR of 2.7—a complicated situation that will be explained more fully later.

There is also a major *geographic* variation in TFRs within American states. In 2002 the *lowest* five states were Vermont (1.60), Maine (1.66), Rhode Island (1.70), Massachusetts (1.71), and New Hampshire (1.73)—mid-European rates. The lowest jurisdiction (as opposed to state) was the District of Columbia at 1.58. The five *highest* states were all Western or Southwestern: Alaska (2.5), Utah (2.54), Arizona (2.36), Texas (2.35), and Idaho (2.28)—higher than many Less Developed Countries.

In all, America's two-child Total Fertility Rate is good—natural and normal. What's astonishing is that this natural and normal rate is abnormal in the rest of the world.

CHAPTER FIVE

America the Exceptional: Immigrant Takers

*"I, personally, have a philosophy that regards America as a
nation with a special race and a special descent. America is made
up of us all, the people of the earth. We have made America. . . .
We are still making America. If our sons go to America in ten
years time they will become Americans. We view America as
belonging to us all. . . . The yellow race is part of America; the
Arabs are part of America; Muslims, the Indians, the Hindus,
the Jews and all nationalities are part of America."*

THE OBSERVATION ABOVE was made by the famous president of
a small nation that has occasionally burst onto the front page. For
a time this president was considered as a very important global
player, albeit not among those nations that viewed America kindly.
Who said it?

Muammar Gaddafi said it, as reported by the U.S. Foreign Broadcast Information Service. I find it unfortunate that a screwball dicta-
tor should get it so right about America while some Americans
actively lobby the government to kill the immigration goose that lays
mostly golden eggs.

It was the economist David Ricardo who in 1817 formalized the
principle of "comparative advantage." The idea is that some nations typically can do some things better than some other nations.

Therefore, in a free trade system, citizens of that nation can effectively market their product or service in the international arena, enriching themselves and acquiring assets with which to buy goods and services from other countries that can produce different goods or services less expensively. For example, New Zealanders sell mutton to the Japanese; they use the proceeds to buy Japanese cars at lower prices than they could produce cars themselves. "Comparative advantage" is a win-win proposition (except when domestic workers lose their jobs for comparative advantage, in which case holy hell erupts, and politicians quaver).

While America has many comparative advantages on the international playing field, I believe the most important one is that we do immigration best. It would be an American tragedy—and a global tragedy—if we were to move toward a seriously restrictionist policy. This is not an idle concern. One of America's leading immigration scholars, a most sensible man, George Borjas, favors cutting immigration in half. America placed heavy restrictions on immigration once before, in the 1920s, and it took forty years before the policy was again liberalized.

Overall, immigration in America has worked out extremely well. That said, it has always been trouble. Even before the United States was formed, Benjamin Franklin complained about too many Germans in America, sticking together in clans within the colonies, still speaking German. When the Irish arrived in the mid-1800s they were greeted with employment signs reading "No Irish Need Apply," and were routinely described as drunks who looked like "gorillas." By some estimates, it took the Irish a century to catch up to median American incomes. (Nomination for best recent book title: Noel Ignatiev's *How the Irish Became White*.) In 1882, America passed a "Chinese Exclusion Act."

The huge immigration wave of the late nineteenth and early twentieth centuries contributed to tumultuous times in America. Immigration was a central issue. Many early social scientists promoted the theory of what is now called "scientific racism," which "proved"—surprise!—that persons from Northwest Europe (like themselves) were biologically superior. Obviously the new immigrants, mostly Jews, Poles, and Italians from Southern and Eastern Europe, were not very smart, and if well-measured they would be found way down on the totem pole of intelligence.

In such a climate the resurgence of the Ku Klux Klan was not necessarily seen as wholly retrograde. The Klan was originally known for its night-riding, cross-burning anti-Negro activity after the Civil War, but it was sparked a second time—notably in the cities—in large measure by anti-immigration sentiment. By the early 1920s the KKK was a far-flung organization. Interestingly, the state with the highest proportion of KKK members was not in the South, it was Indiana. Immigrant Catholics and Jews as well as blacks were the targets of the time.

The Klan may have been generally disreputable but not totally so. In their landmark work of sociology, *Middletown*, published in 1929, Robert and Helen Lynd listed the Klan under the rubric of "social organizations."

And anti-immigration sentiment could be found well into the intellectual mainstream. Consider the views of the former superintendent of the Census Bureau, one Francis Walker, who later became president of MIT. In 1896 he wrote: "The entrance of such vast masses of peasantry, degraded below our utmost conceptions, is a matter which no intelligent patriot can look upon without the gravest apprehension and alarm. They are beaten men from beaten races. They have none of the ideas and aptitudes such as belong to those who were descended from the tribes that met under the oak trees of old Germany to make laws and choose chiefs." (Note to Francis Walker, wherever you are: Germany did not do well in the first half of the twentieth century.)

Fast forward to the late twentieth century. The charts on the following pages show that by high ratios Americans now say it's a good thing that Poles, Italians, Irish, and Jews emigrated to America. But remember that the grandparents and great-grandparents of the respondents were typically the people who thought the ancestors of those wonderful Italians, Irish, Poles, and Jews were nothing more than (as Francis Walker believed) beaten men from beaten races: dagos, Micks, Polacks, and kikes.

(Oscar Handlin of Harvard won the Pulitzer Prize for history with his 1951 book *The Uprooted*. He writes with passion of the wave of

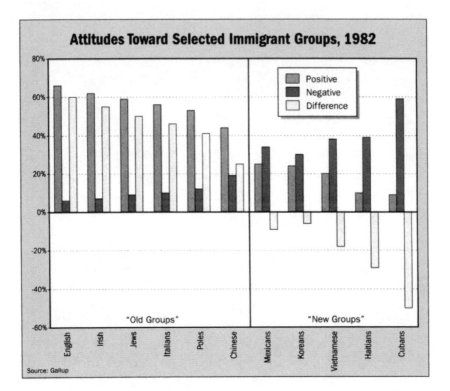

Attitudes Toward Selected Immigrant Groups, 1982

Positive
Negative
Difference

"Old Groups" "New Groups"

English Irish Jews Italians Poles Chinese Mexicans Koreans Vietnamese Haitians Cubans

Source: Gallup

25 million immigrants who arrived in the late nineteenth and early twentieth centuries. He uses Census data to point out that, unlike earlier immigrants, these newcomers were principally of peasant stock. Consider Handlin's words about them: "They discovered a setting that compelled them to improvise and imposed upon them the obligation to act the risky role of individuals. In doing so, they and their children revealed a potentiality for achievement unimaginable in the village. . . . They discovered the glory and the grief of being free.")

As in the past, today it is the newcomers who are seen with disfavor. This time it is Koreans, Cubans, Vietnamese, and Mexicans. But those views change over time too. As the charts show, the newcomer groups scored substantially higher in the 1990s than in the 1980s. Americans may have trouble with newcomers, but by the time the newcomers have been around for a while, attitudes change. The immigration scholar Rita Simon has put it nicely: "The American public tends to look at immigration with rear-facing rose-colored glasses."

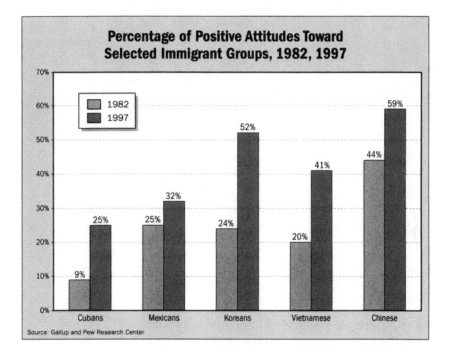

Percentage of Positive Attitudes Toward Selected Immigrant Groups, 1982, 1997

Source: Gallup and Pew Research Center

Anti-immigration activity today is pussycat stuff compared to what went before. There are no night-riders, no arson, no lynchings. Still, the same themes resonate.

BECAUSE IT IS now the country sending the greatest number of immigrants to America, Mexico is at the root of today's anti-immigration argument. It will serve us well to take a closer look at that situation.

The big words tossed around in the argument are "assimilation" and "acculturation." Just beneath that level of discourse is some familiar exclusionary thinking.

It is argued these days—part of what is called the "swamping" argument—that this time the immigration is different. Mexicans, it is said, talk Spanish, not English, and they will never speak English well because their "real" home country is just across that narrow river called the Rio Grande. We are told they go back and forth to Mexico all the time, watch Spanish television and movies, read Spanish newspapers and magazines. As part of a *Reconquista* movement, they really want to set up a nation called "Aztlán," which would make

California and the American Southwest part of Mexico. The new Mexicans, it is said, represent a part of a Third Worlding of America. They are not white, the restrictionists say, they stick out like a sore thumb; and they just keep coming and coming and coming, like beige Energizer bunnies overrunning an already crowded nation, having babies and more babies, sometimes as a way of securing citizenship.

The election for governor of California in a late 2003 recall election was won by Arnold Schwarzenegger, an immigrant. But the state's lieutenant governor, Cruz Bustamante, refused to renounce his collegiate membership in the irredentist Movimiento Estudiantil Chicano de Aztlán, or MEChA—more fodder for anti-immigration sentiment in America.

Pat Buchanan has become the fountainhead of such anti-Mexican sentiment in America these days. What he says is pretty much wrong. The good news is, his bad news is wrong.

As the 2000 Census data trickled out, one item hit the headline jackpot. The census results showed more Hispanics than had been expected and in theory made Hispanics "America's largest minority," surpassing blacks somewhat earlier than had been anticipated. This played into an earlier story which trumpeted that by the year 2050 or thereabouts, America would be "majority nonwhite." Somewhat more technically, it was said that American minorities would constitute a majority. (Some blacks felt this was a blow to their standing and self-esteem. But blacks are much more likely to vote than Latinos, and they wield greater political clout.)

There has, of course, been a major change in American immigration. In 1960 the proportion of Europeans in U.S. immigration was 75 percent. By 1970 (after a more open immigration law was passed in 1965, amending the restrictive 1924 "quota" bill) the percentage of European immigrants was 60 percent. In 1980 it was 37 percent. In 1990 it was 22 percent. In 2000 the proportion of European immigrants was 16 percent. (Data from 2000 comes from the U.S. Census Bureau; data from 1960–1990 comes from Census Bureau Working Paper #29 by Campbell Gibson and Emily Lennon.)

This story of whites being swallowed up by immigrants has been around in one form or another for at least a century, and in its current incarnation for about twenty years. These days, typically, "nonwhite" and/or "minority" has been defined rather rigidly: blacks, Asians, Hispanics, and Native Americans. By an executive order of the president, no one else qualifies for official minority status in many federal programs.

(But what about the Jews? I grew up as a "minority" in an all-Jewish neighborhood—not a ghetto, not segregated, just all-Jewish except for one Italian-American family whose breadwinner owned the local grocery store. How did I end up being counted as a majoritarian Anglo male? I have no problem with it, but I also feel strongly and warmly about being Jewish. And what about the descendants of Italian immigrants? Or, reaching back just a bit further, Irish Americans?)

Here is what the recent immigration numbers look like: In the decade of the 1990s (1991–2000), America admitted more legal immigrants than in any previous decade. According to the Immigration and Naturalization Service, the net total was 9.1 million, not counting illegals. The highest previous decade was almost a full century earlier, 1901–1910, when the total was almost the same, 8.8 million. There are, however, more illegal immigrants entering the United States these days than in days past, thanks in some large part to ease of transportation and easier border crossing.

Buchanan and many others in the anti-immigrant camp say those nine million immigrants per decade will "swamp" American culture, turning us into a chaotic Third World nation. But the assumption is wrongheaded. Look at rates, not absolute numbers. In the 1901–1910 decade those nine million immigrants made up about 1 percent per year (1.04 percent) of the total American population. In the 1990s the nine million immigrants represented only .036 percent of the American population. (America had grown; immigration was about one-third of its earlier rate.) To sense what is happening today, visualize a cocktail party in a hotel ballroom. Many hundreds of people are talking and drinking, ice cubes are clinking and melting, hors d'oeuvres are running low and turning soggy. In walks an immigrant couple from Mexico. Pat Buchanan turns to you and says, "See, they're swamping us."

Or look at it through another lens. Back in 1910, almost 15 percent of Americans were foreign-born. In 1924, America established a restrictive immigration code. By 1970 the number of foreign-born residents had fallen to about 5 percent. At about that time (1965), new, less restrictive immigration laws were enacted. And by 1999 the foreign-born figure had risen to about 10 percent, still only about halfway up the ladder to the previous high-water mark. Nine of ten Americans are born in America, even with all those recent Mexican immigrants, legal and illegal.

Or look at the "foreign stock" data, which until recently was the terminology used by the Census Bureau to designate those Americans born in foreign lands *and* their offspring, even if those offspring had only one foreign-born parent. Back in 1910 the foreign stock of America amounted to 34 percent. A third of the country was of foreign stock, and the heavens did not collapse. America stumbled through the century in pretty good shape. Today the comparable figure is 21 percent.

America can take in more immigrants if it wants to. Should we? In the current amounts, which I consider moderate, I think it should be considered. How so? To begin, immigration is essentially what keeps America growing. Today the typical American woman bears less than the replacement rate of 2.1 children during the course of her fertile years.* As noted earlier, Hispanic fertility rates are the highest of any racial or ethnic group in America, at about 2.7 children per woman. But one reason the Hispanic fertility rate is higher is because the immigration is ongoing, and the immigrant generation has substantially

---

*In 2002 the National Center for Health Statistics announced that for the first time since 1972 the American TFR had climbed above the 2.1 replacement rate. That was data for 2001, reflecting mostly conceptions in 2000, before the recession. It was reported in all the newspapers—for one day. For demographic wonks, that was big news. It broke, or seemed to break, a thirty-year string of American below-replacement TFRs, since 1972. But several months later, in February 2003, the NCHS revised the 2001 numbers to 2.03, below the replacement level—more than three decades and counting. No newspaper coverage.

What happened? In the first instance, the NCHS used 2001 population estimates projected from the 1990 Census, which did not fully account for subsequent immigration in the 1990s. When the 2000 Census data appeared, the estimates more accurately reflected the size and growth of the Hispanic population. That increased the number of Hispanics while the number of Hispanic births remained constant. Raise the denominator, don't raise the numerator—and lower the Total Fertility Rate. The corrected 2001 Hispanic TFR was 2.7 children per woman instead of the 3.2 originally reported—16 percent lower, a rather important difference.

higher fertility than its offspring, just as other first-generation Americans did in earlier times.

Were there no Hispanics in America, the United States would in theory sooner or later experience population loss, undoubtedly later. The Medium Variant of the most recent Census Bureau projection posits that American population will grow from 282 million in 2000 to 420 million in 2050, including expected immigration. Without immigration the growth would be to about 330 million, on the way to slow population growth, then no population growth.

The difference between a continuation of current immigration trends or a cutoff of immigration is about 90 million people, an amount more than the entire population of Germany. But this population growth in America is by no means a Mexican phenomenon. Only about a fifth (22 percent) of legal immigrants to America come from Mexico. A thumbnail estimate that would include illegals might boost that to 25 to 30 percent. (Remember, illegals come to America from other places too, like Ireland, Israel, the Philippines, Poland, and China.) Moreover, the annual number of Mexican immigrants will almost certainly shrink over the intermediate to long term. As mentioned earlier, the TFR in Mexico has diminished from 6.5 children per woman in the early 1970s to about replacement level now, according to Mexican demographers who say the UN data are slow in picking up the fast drop in the Mexican TFR. The decline, say these demographers, shows no signs of stopping. That will lower the supply side of the Mexican immigration equation.

California is seen as the test tube of a tan America. But often forgotten in the argument is the true demography of the Golden State. Aside from almost twenty million "Anglos," California has a wide variety of non-Hispanic immigrant groups, each with significant numbers. These include Koreans, Filipinos, Chinese, Japanese, Khmer, Russian Jews, Iranians, and Thai, to name just a few. They didn't come from Mexico; they didn't come to be part of a reconquered Aztlán, speaking Spanish. They came to America, and they want their children to speak English.

And, by the way, just as there is some Mexicanization of America, so too is there plenty of Americanization going on in Mexico. In Monterrey the fans root for the Dallas Cowboys and worry that

American movies and television shows are corrupting their youth. (Just as Anglos in Dallas root and worry about the same things.) Moreover, there are a growing number of U.S. citizens, mostly seniors, mostly Anglos, who are relocating to Mexico, a land of low dollar-denominated costs, where a dollar can buy plentiful personal services. Soon perhaps Mexicans will be claiming that Americans are different from other immigrants, that they often travel home, that they continue to speak English.

Michael Barone's book *The New Americans* puts forth an interesting theory: Mexican immigrants are following the course of earlier Italian immigration, with relatively slow educational progress and mild income growth. Asian immigrants, Barone says, follow the Jewish pattern, with fast educational upgrading and good incomes. American blacks (typically, says Barone, from an "immigrant" background in the rural South) follow a pattern akin to Irish immigration—slow assimilation and relatively low wages. But in all cases the movement is ascendant. Different immigrant groups do indeed follow different patterns of socio-economic advancement and acculturation. With all that, a sizable and growing segment of Mexican Americans, like Italians before them, are doing pretty well economically.

But American history tells us that most all will Americanize sooner or later. A 1998 California initiative (Proposition 227) repealed California's bilingual education programs by a wide margin. Proponents maintained that bilingual instruction was preventing some Latino students from rapid advancement in English-language proficiency. This grew out of a movement of Latina mothers who were fed up by a bilingual bureaucracy. Originally, polls showed more than two-thirds of the Latino voters supported the proposition. Even after much money was spent by opponents to paint the proposal as an anti-Hispanic slam, almost half the Hispanic voters supported the initiative.

The word is out in Hispanic communities: Latina mothers tell their children, with no intent to disparage the Spanish language in any way, that "Spanish is the language of busboys." They stress a commonsense notion: in America you have to speak English to get ahead.

More on Mexico, our surrogate state for the general condition of immigration in the United States today:

* Third World? Mexico's per capita income is above $5,000. It now has "investment grade" bond status. Mexico is a member of the Organization for Economic Cooperation and Development, the First World economic club. It is a real if imperfect democracy, with an opposition party president. In the last six years the Mexican economy grew substantially faster per capita than did that of the United States: 3.0 percent versus 2.2 percent.

* Invasion? How many invaders compete to mow the lawns and wash the dishes of those they have conquered? We tend to forget that America needs poor immigrants as well as well-to-do ones. And we forget too that historically the progeny of the busboys move up the socioeconomic ladder. It's happening with Mexican-American immigrants.

* Assimilation? By the third generation just about all Mexican Americans speak English, and Mexican-born grandparents often complain that their grandchildren speak no Spanish, a familiar complaint in the history of American immigration.

* Not Western? Scholars say the *padrones* of Latin America, the hegemonic roots of the culture, are language and religion. The languages in the Hispanic case are Spanish or Portuguese—European tongues. The basic religion is Catholic, with growing evangelical Protestant sects—Christians just like most Americans.

* Mexican Americans serve disproportionately in America's armed services. Proportionate to their numbers in the military, they have won the most medals for gallantry in combat.

* The sore thumb argument is losing potency. "Exogamy" is the uptown word for "intermarriage." And despite all the talk of the balkanization, Mexican Americans are intermarrying in high numbers. Once again the people are creating demography, and it looks like the putatively outmoded notion of the "melting pot."

How much exogamy? Census data from 1990 shows that 64 percent of Asians in the United States married outside their race or ethnic group. The rate for all Hispanics was 37 percent, but experts believe that the rate climbs with the second and third generation. The rate also remains somewhat low because the Hispanic population is regularly replenished by newcomers. The black intermarriage rate is much lower but is climbing at a very fast rate, from about 3 percent in 1980, to 5 percent in 1990, and 9 percent in 1998.

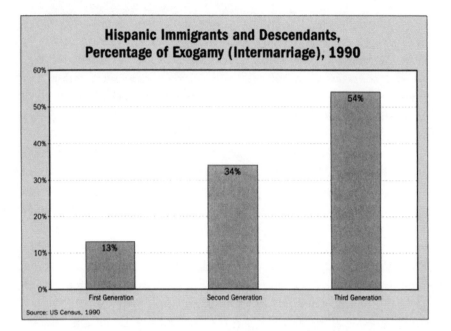

Hispanic Immigrants and Descendants, Percentage of Exogamy (Intermarriage), 1990

Source: US Census, 1990

Of course, no large immigration will be without troubles. Mexican Americans have higher crime rates than the American average but lower than the African-American rate. On the other hand, Mexican-American young people are more likely to drop out of high school than are blacks.

Seen up close, the Mexican immigration can get very personal. Here are excerpts from a letter I received after the *Think Tank* program with Pat Buchanan in 2002:

> Wattenberg should get out of his Ivory Tower and see what is really happening to this country. . . . As a Catholic growing up in Chicago, I have seen the Irish, Poles, Germans, Lithuanians, Greeks, Italians, etc. pushed out of neighborhood after neighborhood by Latinos who actually hate the white "gringos." My own neighborhood is a Spanish ghetto of high crime and degraded property values. The Europeans who came here at the turn of the century were proud to become Americans, learn the English language and contribute to the growth and economy of a great America. They had a respect for education and worked hard

to be an AMERICAN. The new immigrant Mexicans have overrun this country with their language and their culture: everything has to be bilingual in favor of Spanish. We didn't see German/English, Lithuanian/English, Italian/English overrun our telephone systems, advertising, even simple package directions. Every nationality that has come to this country, except the Mexicans, assimilates. Even Muslim Arabs who are new to the Chicago area act and live like Americans, and yes, even have their children speak English, more than Mexicans who have resided here longer.

And the resentment against immigration is not just against Mexicans. I recall with some vividness how I stumbled upon Wattenberg's First Law of book writing: "Do the talk shows, *then* write the book."

I had written a book entitled *The First Universal Nation*, published in 1991. In it I carefully explained why legal immigration is good for America, and why I believed we should moderately raise our immigration levels. Then I did the call-in talk shows. I traveled to several cities, sometimes doing five or more television and radio call-in programs in a day. After I returned from the tour I did about fifty talk show "phoners" from my desk in Washington, connected with people from across the country.

About half the callers agreed with me. What a swell fellow I was, they burbled, I understood what made America great, and weren't we all descended from immigrants, anyway? Immigration was a glory (and that included Latinos).

The other half of the callers thought I was a lout, or worse. A Pakistani neighbor threw garbage out the window of the apartment house. Los Angeles was turning into a Third World city. Spanish was the new language of Miami, and people who grew up there in pre-Castro days didn't like it one bit. The Cuban immigrants were stealing our country from us.

The calls didn't change my mind about immigration, but they would have changed the tone of the book—for the better—had I understood the depth of anti-immigrant feeling that still runs deep among many Americans.

In any event, America should get much tougher and smarter about illegal immigrants. Why? The first reason is that they are illegal. Tens of millions of people in the world seek admission to America. Jumping the queue breaks down the system of law. That was a sensible policy before the 9/11 massacre; now it is imperative, with particular scrutiny of persons from Muslim nations that are regarded as terrorist havens—even if the Arab Americans observed by the Chicago correspondent to *Think Tank* believes they're swell fellows, which they probably are. The trouble is, no major modern country has done a good job of curtailing illegal immigration. The only solution will be long term as population falls everywhere and the economic gap between less developed and more developed nations narrows.

IN 1991 the historian Arthur Schlesinger looked around him and wrote a book called *The Disuniting of America*. He asked: Are we too pluribus and not enough unum? It was the right question. But I believe that on balance the blending is winning out. It was an issue a century ago too. Consider Israel Zangwill's 1908 play *The Melting Pot*, which had the longest run on Broadway of any play to that day. The plot line is elemental. The son of a cossack officer emigrates to America. He falls in love with a Jewish girl. It turns out that the cossack officer had been an active participant in the Russian pogroms that had killed the girl's father. The climactic moment comes when the son says this:

> America is God's crucible, the great melting pot, where all the
> races of Europe are melting and reforming. Here you stand,
> good folks, and your fifty groups with your fifty languages and
> histories, and your fifty blood hatreds and rivalries, a fig for
> your feuds and vendettas. Germans and Frenchmen, Irishmen
> and Englishmen, Jews and Russians, in the crucible with you all.
> God is making the American.

Half a century after Zangwill's play, the Harvard scholars Daniel P. Moynihan and Nathan Glazer questioned the hallowed idea in their landmark book of ethnic sociology, *Beyond the Melting Pot* (1964). Their work covered Irish, Jews, Italians, blacks, and Puerto Ricans. Their general view was that there was less melting going on than supposed. Old-country cultures had a way of hanging on. (And Pat Moynihan used to chortle that Zangwill later emigrated to Palestine.)

But they hang on for only so long. The great Yiddish daily newspapers (center left, left, and very left) have disappeared. The old ethnic neighborhoods dissolve. The churches and synagogues move to the suburbs. Tony Soprano's parents surely lived on Mulberry Street in New York City, not in suburban New Jersey where Tony hangs his hat and other things. Many blacks in Northeast D.C. have moved to suburban Prince George's County, a relatively well-to-do jurisdiction of 816,000 where 63 percent are black. Meanwhile, gentrifying whites are moving back into D.C., and within a decade or two blacks may no longer be a majority in the city. This is viewed with alarm by some in the black community, who believe it is part of "The Plan" of whites and the business community to take away the majority status of blacks in the nation's capital. I don't believe it. It's just what keeps on happening in America over and over again.

Assimilation is in the saddle. At colleges with fraternities, some Jewish students belong to Jewish fraternities, some do not. Jewish fraternities are substantially less popular than they used to be; Jewish students now often join Gentile fraternities; Gentiles join Jewish fraternities. There used to be great pride among Jews, almost proprietary in nature, of a "Jewish seat" on the U.S. Supreme Court. Then for a while there were no Jewish justices on the Court, and no one seemed to care. In recent years there have been two Jewish justices, Stephen Breyer and Ruth Bader Ginsburg, and still no one in the Jewish community seems to care. The National Jewish Population Survey, 2000–2001, reports that 54 percent of Jews marry outside their faith, up from 52 percent in 1990. (This data prompts a complex argument, as does the true Jewish TFR in America.)

Perhaps "melting pot" is too harsh a metaphor for this time. Molten steel and iron pouring from huge buckets is so twentieth century. During the high point of the separatist multi-culti movement, other metaphors were suggested: "mosaic" and "salad bowl" each trying to emphasize the remaining differences in America. There are plenty, of course.

I see the process as in a slow-running and not fully efficient blender. That household appliance takes vegetables and fruits from all over the world and creates blends. It does not suggest as harsh a process as "melting pot." Sometimes the results look like Derek Jeter, with one white parent, one black parent, and an arm like a rifle. In the next Census, what box will be ticked for the child of Andrei Agassi (Iranian American) and Steffi Graf (German)? American baseball was once all white, then with many blacks, and now with a heavy Latino component as well. The three single-season major league home run leaders reflect this reality: Barry Bonds, Mark McGwire, and Sammy Sosa.

Israel Zangwill, meet Muammar Gaddafi.

CHAPTER SIX

The Culture of Alarmism

HERE WE SHOULD PAUSE for a moment and ask some questions. First, how good is that UNPD data? The UN demographers are excellent scholars and, near as I can see, do their work very well. They are knowledgeable and cordial. They have been prompt in their dealing with me on this book. I thank them not only in the acknowledgments but right here as well.

Their highlight publication, which appears every two years, is the invaluable *World Population Prospects*. It describes, first, the past (though, in truth, the actual population of Togo in 1955 may not be regarded as a precise number), and, second, estimates the present. When it makes projections about the future, that, as you might imagine, is a problem. In its most-cited set of projections, the UN provides estimates out to the year 2050. That sounds far away, but it is a year when many adults alive today will still be with us. Recall, the UNPD provides three alternative projection scenarios labeled "High," "Medium," and "Low," which it publicizes, and a fourth one, the barely mentioned but very important "Constant-Fertility Variant."

The UNPD itself categorically states that no one projection is more valid than another. But put yourself in the spot of, say, an Associated Press reporter who just got an assignment to write a thousand-word story summarizing global population growth as reported by a just-published edition of *World Population Prospects*. Which "equally" descriptive word would you use in your story, "high," "medium," "low," or "Constant-Fertility Variant"?

"Medium," of course. Even the UN regularly emphasizes "Medium" despite its avowal of neutrality among the major assumptions. Moreover, the differentials between the numbers carry truly enormous leverage. For example, the global difference between a Total Fertility Rate of "medium" and "low" in India is 290 million never-born persons in 2050, roughly the size of the United States today. To oversimplify a bit, that huge difference comes about if one projects that India reaches its 1.85 replacement rate about fifteen years earlier than scheduled under the "Medium" set of projections. That yields fewer potential mothers, and fewer people.

There is an argument about whether "Medium," as presently calculated, is the most likely assumption upon which to base future planning or general thinking about the state of the world. My own view is that "Medium" is overstated, and many demographers share that view. As we have seen, as fertility fell everywhere, the UN itself changed its base goal TFR from 2.11 to 1.85. That act moved its "Medium" projections toward the downside. (I don't know any demographers who think the "High" set of assumptions is where we're headed. And it is interesting to note that even under the "High" assumptions, fertility rates are projected to fall.)

Is this statistical argument important? Somewhat. If the "Medium" projection data overstate fertility, they consequently overstate the number of people on the planet in the future. The "Medium" variant numbers have served as the bedrock for the whole notion of population growth rising by big numbers. They connote demographic danger, a notion that may have been valuable for a while but is becoming less valid with each passing day.

One note of importance: even if the "Medium" projection data were not overstated, the general conclusions in this book are sound and solid.

Just what is "Medium"? Until the publication of the 2002 data, the UNPD "Medium" scenario took every modern nation with a TFR below 2.1 children per woman and by statistical fiat sloped it upward toward 2.1 by 2050. Nations above the replacement level were sloped downward to 2.1.

Now the UN projects that the TFR will fall to 1.85. Recall that every single developed nation—all of Europe, Japan, the United

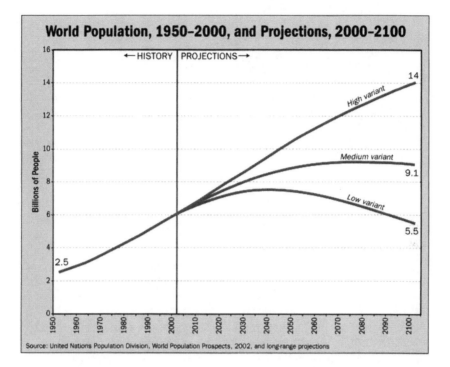

World Population, 1950–2000, and Projections, 2000–2100

← HISTORY | PROJECTIONS →

High variant — 14

Medium variant — 9.1

Low variant — 5.5

2.5

Billions of People

Source: United Nations Population Division, World Population Prospects, 2002, and long-range projections

States, Canada, Australia—is currently in that subreplacement status, and almost all of them have been there for many decades. Yet for most modern countries the new UN projections will *raise* the TFR for the next fifty-year cycle. Why?

There are two basic ways of measuring Total Fertility Rates. The UN bases its projections on the "cohort" measurement, that is, by adding up all the children born during a woman's childbearing years (the calculation is that women are fertile from ages 15 to 44). *It measures what has already happened.* No one is arguing that fertility in the 1970s and 1980s was not higher than it is now. Those high rates provided more potential mothers today, and more people for a few more decades, even if current fertility stays very low. A forty-four-year-old in the year 2000 was of childbearing age as early as 1971,* when Total Fertility Rates were near their all-time high. Then those TFRs declined in the following years but remained at quite high levels. Naturally, if that "completed fertility" measurement is projected

*44 minus 15 equals 29, subtracted from 2000 years equals 1971.

into the future it will show more people than a measurement that uses the current much lower fertility rates.

The other way to measure Total Fertility Rates is the "period" measure. The period rate produces a portrait of what is happening *now*, not in 1970 or 1980. The theory rests on the idea that women in given age cohorts today will continue to have babies at that same rate into the future. That yields lower population totals.

In any event, the difference in the two approaches adds up to .1 to .2 children more (cohort) or less (period). It makes for a good argument in demographic circles, and it has important long-range implications, but it is not massive in its effect.

My own view is somewhat different. I think it is more logical to allow the above-replacement rate nations continue to sink, just as the UN projects. These are the Less Developed Countries, whose fertility rates have been rapidly falling for half a century.

But for nations already well under replacement, I think it is appropriate to use the "Constant-Fertility Variant." That method recall keeps the low TFRs of modern countries *just where they are now.* After all, until we know that change has happened (up or down) or that there is good reason to expect that change will happen (up or down), we should stick with what now prevails.

Ironically, for a variety of technical and since-abandoned UNPD demographic projection rules, Europe records a somewhat larger population under the momentous new 1.85 TFR standard than it did under the old TFR rules. Under the new way of calculating, Europe falls from 728 million to 632 million people from 2000 to 2050, a total decline of 96 million people—an enormous drop. But under the old calculation, Europe fell from 727 million to 603 million, a loss of 124 million people, or about the population of Japan today.

Similarly, Germany would have lost 11 million people by 2050 under the old rules, and only 3 million in 2050 under the new rules. Of course the Germans must be concerned that the number of their residents over eighty years of age will have grown from 3.5 percent to 11.7 percent during that time, and that those people expect their pensions—on time, in the right amount, with no political tricks attached.

All this happens because for the very low fertility countries, the TFR of 1.85 children per woman represents a greater increase than had previously been calculated under the old and complicated UN technical projection rules. In fact, those who believe in a "second demographic transition," to be described later, display formulas indicating that no such increase is in the offing. Their calculations become complicated, but the gist of them is that if TFRs in Europe do not change (using the C-F Variant), Europe's population will fall to 597 million, a decline of 131 million people, almost half the size of the United States. Under any assumption, Europe's population is shrinking markedly.

Moreover the new 1.85 rules do not allow for a further decline in existing current fertility for low-fertility nations. Might not the United Kingdom's TFR fall below its current 1.6 TFR? After all, fertility has been falling in the UK. Nor will the UN projection rules allow any Less Developed Country to fall below 1.85, even though many have already done so. As mentioned, South Korea, for example, is now at 1.17—but the new rules say it must rise to 1.85.

Something else on the horizon will lower population estimates. Since 1994, about a decade ago, the UNPD has been using 2050 as the end of its basic projections. In a time of expected falling fertility (like now), the farther out the projection, the lower the population. Appropriately, the UN plans new projections, possibly in 2006 or 2008, when the end-year projection will move forward toward 2075. When those projections are published, further attention will be drawn to the remarkable demographic era in which we live.

For the far-out future, these statistics have enormous leverage. Suppose the new UN level of 1.85 children per woman holds until the year 2300. In that event, global population would fall from a high of about 9 billion to 2.3 billion people! Of course, if replacement is reached well before 2300, that 2.3 billion figure would be much higher—about 9 billion. Sooner or later, everyone agrees, global fertility will have to climb back to replacement level. If not, the human species will not survive. But when?

IF THE UN POPULATION NUMBERS are overstated, why might that be so? I do not know with certainty, but I have some questions that I believe deserve consideration. My starting point is that the general ambience of an organization has an influence, quite often un-witting, on its policies.

One possible ambient reason for the earlier 2.1 high bias of the "Medium" scenario for the modern nations is that UN member nations do not like the idea of "going out of business," a phrase demographers play around with. It riles the natives. In the past, Italians, Greeks, Spaniards, Russians, and Germans have not wished to hear that their peoples are dwindling, caught in a downward spiral such as the world has never seen before. They don't like to lose political heft. Such data also lead to political problems that have been easier to ignore than to confront. For example, lots of old people and relatively few younger people means that nations cannot meet their pension obligations without increasing taxes or lowering benefits. Politicians heard the nervousness of their constituents and promised they would not raise taxes or lower benefits to cover pension costs. For the UN, it was easier to stick with that earlier 2.1 figure and say it would all work out.

(American politicians are not immune. In the summer of 1989, Dan Rostenkowski, chairman of the House Ways and Means Committee, successfully endorsed mandatory "catastrophic" health coverage for Medicare recipients, which would cost subscribers $800 to $1,050 per year. Chased by fifty seniors yelling "Coward," "Recall," and "Impeach," Rostenkowski ran to his car to get away from the irate mob. The law was soon struck from the books, but the TV pictures of the event left a lasting message to elected office holders: Don't take money away from seniors.)

I doubt that any European diplomat has gone directly to the professional demographers at the UN's Population Division and said, "Get those numbers up." The UN demographers would not respond to such pressure. But when the UN Population Division in 2000 issued a document entitled "Replacement Migration," showing that the numbers of immigrants necessary for the European nations to keep their numbers up would be both enormous and implausible, the report struck a nerve on the continent. After the headlines and the news programs had their run with it, recall that the quite august European Union told the UNPD not to do it again.

Speaking of organizational ambience, the UN has a clear mind-set regarding family planning and environmentalism. A large and separate agency that deals with the reduction of population growth, the United Nations Population Fund (with the acronym UNFPA, for United Nations Fund for Population Activities), is never to be confused with the professional demographers at the UN Population Division. I agree with the UNFPA's general goals, though they routinely exaggerate and misuse demographic data, often with an anti-American slant. I have no problem with the UN offering family-planning funds to governments, providing its execution is noncoercive, as it was briefly in India and for decades in China. I have little problem with the UN providing aid to family-planning organizations that offer abortion counseling.*

But I have a major problem when public agencies, like the UNFPA, claim demographic expertise and exaggerate demographic situations using crafted data and rhetoric aimed at the unwitting who must make decisions. In the 1990s, well after the plunge in fertility rates, there was a general budget cutback at the UN. The UNFPA did not like the idea of lower funding for its programs, and issued press releases making the foolish case that population would go back *up* unless its funds were restored.

And the agency is still at it. Their March 2004 press release concerning a UN meeting in Chile of the Economic Commission for Latin America and the Caribbean (ECLAT) declares that of the forty nations attending, "The United States was the only country to disagree with a declaration linking poverty eradication to greater access to services for family planning, safe motherhood and HIV/AIDS protection." It does not mention that the central reason for U.S. objections

---

*Of course, abortion has become a highly politicized matter. Its resolution in UN matters has not worked out badly. When a Republican wins the presidency, the American UN delegation stipulates that American money may not be used for UN-funded institutions that deal with abortion. When a Democratic president is elected, the policy is reversed. What is not generally realized is that when U.S. abortion monies are "cut" under Republicans, the *total* amount of U.S. funding for UN international family planning has not been reduced, only *redirected* to organizations that do not provide legal abortion or abortion counseling. Under either American party, U.S. funds go for some form of family-planning.

was its anti-abortion position, nor that the U.S. contribution to UN family-planning programs has not been cut but only redirected.

Family planning has played an important role in helping families plan their childbearing. But the very idea that family planning alone, and specifically funds offered by the UNFPA, has been the crucial element in reduced fertility does not hold up to scrutiny. Many aspects of low fertility have little to do with official or UN or nongovernmental family-planning programs. For example, the move from farms to cities has occurred throughout the world and is clearly related to lower fertility.

Needless to say, family planning groups like International Planned Parenthood are also prone to exaggeration. So too are environmental activist groups and many important foundations. For the most part, the idea has been not to upset the ostrich cart.

For the UNFPA and the private groups that work with them keeping the green pot boiling, it was an advantage to keep that Medium Variant high. That keeps population up and makes alarmism easier.

I am not a UN hater. The international organization does good work in many social and humanitarian fields and in many areas of the world. It deals with certain political and military situations that could not be well handled without the flag and imprimatur of an international organization. But it would be naive to think that the UN does not have its own code and its own politics.

This is the same organizational culture that declared "Zionism is racism"; that twice fudged and vastly exaggerated the summary document of a careful scientific report on global warming; that apologized for the Chinese practice of forced abortion; that tolerated official anti-Semitic filth at Durban in 2001; that championed a "new world information order" that would have obligated all the world's media outlets to publish only "news" approved by their governments.

Population alarmism has always been a bedrock issue in the environmental cause. At the root of most every environmental argument—pollution, water, global warming, strip malls—is that there are "too many people." If only there weren't so many people, our environmental problems would be so much easier to deal with.

Population alarmism is powered by some sturdy engines of recent intellectual thought. The family-planning movement has a long history in America, going back at least to the high-profile activity of Margaret Sanger in the early twentieth century. Mrs. Sanger had three children of her own and lived in an American nation where the Total Fertility Rate was closer to four than to three. Her basic case made good sense, and by my lights still does. People everywhere should be able to control their own fertility. They should have access to contraception and access to the know-how to use contraception. With some real merit, these fairly simple ideas became the causes of most governments around the world while their advocates became the recipients of much philanthropic largesse.

But the family-planning movement also had a dark side. It emerged at a time when the idea of eugenics had gained at least semi-scientific standing. If, as eugenicists believed, the world was being overrun by poor, ignorant, and dark-skinned people, family planning would minimize the threat.

The fear of "too many people," usually linked with "too little food," goes back to antiquity. Joseph made his reputation with the pharaoh by looking ahead, seeing a famine, and storing grain lest the people starve. Thomas Malthus in 1798 set the benchmark for modern demographics, noting that the food supply grew arithmetically while population grew geometrically, leading therefore to catastrophe. Many modern environmental thinkers have picked up the general Malthusian idea, if not its specifics. The first line of Paul Ehrlich's 1968 book *The Population Bomb* read this way: "The battle to feed humanity is over." He predicted famines in the 1970s where "hundreds of millions will starve to death in spite of any crash programs." At best, he predicted, America and Europe would require "mild" food rationing.

The famines never happened, for several reasons. Population did grow, but people became better fed as new agricultural technology took hold. This has been clearly measured by caloric intake data from the UN Food and Agriculture Organization (plus 27 percent per capita since 1963). Moreover, there is a political dimension to this matter: the scholar Amartya Sen, of Harvard and Cambridge, makes the powerful point that no famine has occurred in a democratic country. These days famine has become a political and military tool.

Later on, "food" became transmogrified into "resources," as in "We're running out of resources." This notion, too, has problems.

After all, "renewable" resources are—renewable. "Nonrenewable" resources have proved to be far more extensive than imagined. (We've been "running out of oil" for more than a hundred years.) And those nonrenewable resources seem to be invariably "substitutable." That is, should we "run out" of copper there are dozens of other conductors, including fiber optics, made from glass, which is made from sand, of which there is plenty.

Time after time the population alarmists have been proved wrong. But macro-environmentalism has a quasi-religious component to it. At one point *Time* magazine went so far as to declare that environmental problems could not be objectively reported. It was so clear that environmental catastrophe, triggered by population growth, was over the horizon that *Time*'s editors and writers had to take arms in the fight. In a fine bit of irony, some years later Time Inc. bought CNN, whose founder Ted Turner and his then-wife Jane Fonda were even more extreme on environmental matters than *Time* was.

And there is always something new in the deck. After decades of preaching that the world is about to enter a cooling cycle, the too-many-people argument is now moved forward by the specter of global warming, and it is greenhouse gases produced by human beings that are the culprits to be publicized. (No serious scientists argue that there won't be some warming; the question is how much, and how much harm, if any, it will cause.)

Interestingly, the original UN study on global warming based its findings on a forthcoming world population of 11.5 billion. Since then it has become apparent that an 8.5 billion peak is much more likely than 11.5 billion. But the old number stayed in use long after its time because it made the alarmist numbers more alarming. The original UN-sponsored statement on the matter was far less than categorical, though it was portrayed that way. The document, put out by the Intergovernmental Panel on Climate Change, said: "The *balance* of evidence *suggests* that there is a *discernable* human influence on global climate" (my italics).

WHICH SCENARIO do you believe? I believe that as the LDC nations modernize, they will become more modern. Therefore fertility in those regions will continue to fall, just as they have fallen for the last forty years. In the modern world I don't know what will happen, because rates seem so low they can hardly fall further. But few thought that modern rates would fall as far as they already have. When I wrote *The Birth Dearth* in the mid-1980s, European fertility was 1.83. It is now 1.38. Accordingly, while I believe the so-called "Low" projection may be too low, I believe it should be somewhat lower than what will happen in the "Medium" assumption.

Aside from the technicalities—which happen to be very important—there are several critical points upon which there is general agreement: (1) Fertility in the modern nations has fallen very, very low. (2) LDC fertility is falling rapidly from an originally high base and will no doubt continue to fall for many decades. And (3) The world will have a lower total population than previously assumed.

CHAPTER SEVEN

Why?

DO WE KNOW *why* fertility rates have declined so rapidly, every-where? Some standard correlations still hold true, but there are also some new conjectures. Together they portend a continued drop in the number of children per woman. This is true despite some heartening progress in the field of fertility enhancement. Here are some factors, plus and minus, that affect the situation.

Farm to city. In 1900 there were 5.7 million farm operators in America. By the year 2000 the number had fallen below 2 million in a nation whose population had grown by four times. An agricul-tural revolution—better seeds, fertilizers, irrigation, machines, and so on—had driven down farm prices so as to make it impossible for many farmers to make a living off the land. And so they moved to ur-ban surroundings. In 1900 well over half the American population lived in rural areas. In 2000 the figure was 21 percent.

A similar move to urban areas has occurred around the world, very noticeably in the Less Developed Countries during the last few decades. From 1960 to 2000 the Nigerian urban population climbed from 14 to 44 percent. In Mexico the rate rose from 51 to 74 percent. In Cameroon from 14 to 49 percent. In South Korea from 28 to 82 percent. "Mega-cities" of ten million and more have blossomed in many parts of the world.*

*In 2001, according to the UN's "World Urbanization Prospects," there were 17 "urban agglomerations" (cities and their suburbs) of 10 million people or more. In rank order they were: Tokyo, 27 million; Sao Paulo, 18 million; Mexico City, 18

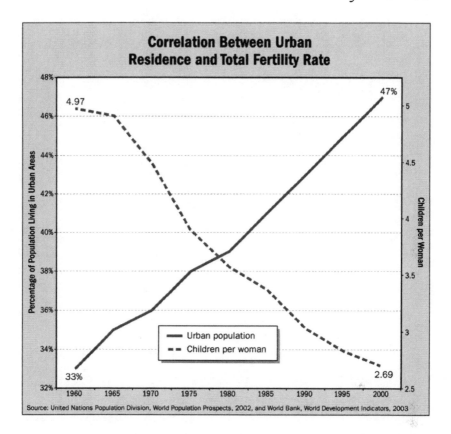

Correlation Between Urban Residence and Total Fertility Rate

Source: United Nations Population Division, World Population Prospects, 2002, and World Bank, World Development Indicators, 2003

On a farm, a child is often regarded as an extra worker to help in agricultural production, starting at a young age. In an urban surrounding, a child is typically a cost, not a benefit. As the trend toward urban movement continues, fertility should continue to fall.

Education for women; working women. The education of women and the entry of women in the work force are also clearly trends in motion, most everywhere. In America in 1947, more than twice as many men went to college as did women. Today more women go to college in America than do men. (The crossover year was 1979.)

In the Less Developed Countries, similar trends can be found, albeit from lower educational levels. In the last decades of the twentieth

million; New York City, 17 million; Bombay, 17 million; Los Angeles, 13 million; Calcutta, 13 million; Dacca, 13 million; New Delhi, 13 million; Shanghai, 13 million; Buenos Aires, 12 million; Jakarta, 11 million; Osaka, 11 million; Beijing, 11 million; Rio de Janeiro, 11 million; Karachi, 10 million; and Manila, 10 million.

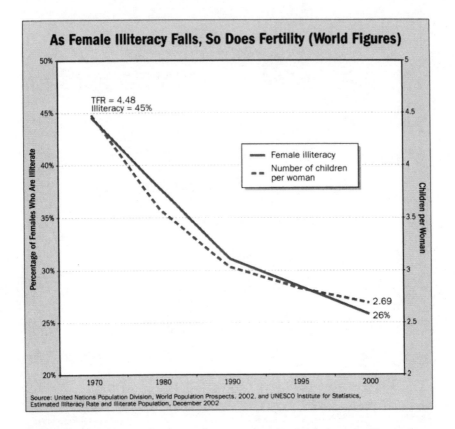

As Female Illiteracy Falls, So Does Fertility (World Figures)

TFR = 4.48
Illiteracy = 45%

— Female illiteracy
- - - Number of children per woman

2.69
26%

Percentage of Females Who Are Illiterate

Children per Woman

1970   1980   1990   1995   2000

Source: United Nations Population Division, World Population Prospects, 2002, and UNESCO Institute for Statistics, Estimated Illiteracy Rate and Illiterate Population, December 2002

century, secondary education for women climbed sharply. For example, from 1970 to 2000 the Egyptian rate went from 15 percent to 77 percent.

Some of the LDC numbers are still very low, but the "illiteracy rate" data is more encouraging. Literacy is achieved in primary school. In Malaysia, from 1970 to 2000, the illiteracy rate fell from 42 to 13 percent. In Mexico from 27 to 9 percent. In Indonesia from 44 to 13 percent.

In America, among women of childbearing age, the proportion of women in the labor force increased from 34 to 60 percent in the second half of the twentieth century. Similar trends are apparent in European countries.

Long-established correlations have shown that literate women, who work in the paid labor force, have fewer children. It takes time to raise a child. More education, more work, lower fertility.

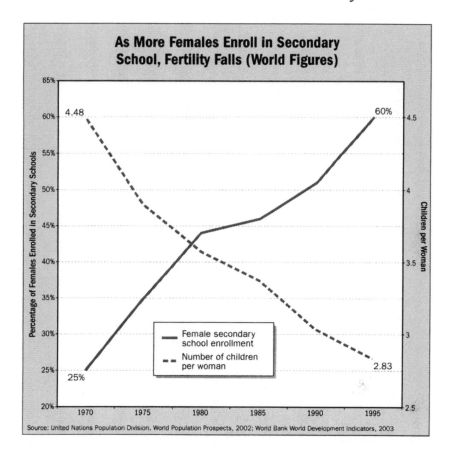

As More Females Enroll in Secondary School, Fertility Falls (World Figures)

Source: United Nations Population Division, World Population Prospects, 2002; World Bank World Development Indicators, 2003

Abortion. In the United States in 1990 there were 1.6 million abortions, the greatest number ever. By the year 2000 the number had fallen to 1.3 million. While I applaud the reduction, I find the current rate a particularly tragic situation when so many parents are trying to adopt and are having great difficulty doing so. Worldwide, in 1995, there were 45.5 million abortions. Of those, 25.6 million were legal and 19.9 million illegal.*

I am barely pro-choice, but I have never forgotten the early days of the feminist movement when abortion activists took out newspaper ads that sounded to me like bragging about having abortions. That distressed me. As President Clinton stressed: keep it rare.

*Source: Alan Guttmacher Institute.

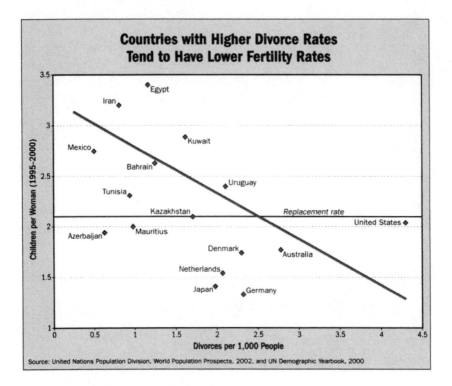

In attitude, the Protestant and Catholic pro-choice rates are about equal—56 percent of Protestants and 59 percent of Catholics say abortion should be "legal in all cases" and "legal in most cases," results within the margin of error. The Jewish rate is 91 percent.*

Divorce. In 1960, in America, the rate of divorce was 2.2 per 1,000 population. It climbed to 5.2 in 1980. By 1998 it had fallen to 4.3. High divorce rates tend to lower fertility.

Contraception. Not only has the use of contraception increased in the United States in recent times, but there has been a shift to more effective methods of birth control. In the 1960s "the pill" and male and female sterilizations were popular. Later, by the 1990s, longer-acting hormonal methods, like Norplant and injectable Depo-Provera, showed increased usage.

*Source: Voter News Service, a consortium of ABC News, the Associated Press, CBS News, CNN, Fox News, and NBC News.

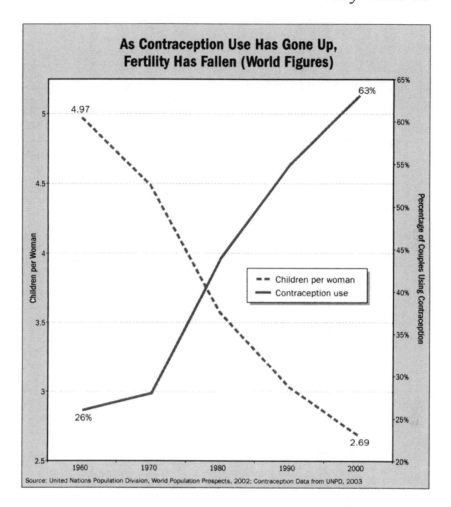

As Contraception Use Has Gone Up, Fertility Has Fallen (World Figures)

Source: United Nations Population Division, World Population Prospects, 2002; Contraception Data from UNPD, 2003

A 1965 survey of currently married American women showed 64 percent using some form of contraception. In 1995 the figure was 76 percent. From 1993 to 2002 the rate of employer-provided health plans covering a wide range of contraceptive choices climbed from 28 percent to 86 percent, according to parallel studies of the Alan Guttmacher Institute. Similar data are to be found worldwide.

Globally, UN data from 2001 show that 61 percent of the more than 1 billion married or in-union women of reproductive age are using contraception. Rates have increased substantially in the last decade. In December 2003 two advisory committees to the U.S. Food and Drug Administration voted 23 to 4 to allow a "morning-after" pill to be marketed over the counter rather than by prescription. The pill can reduce the chance of pregnancy by 89 percent if used within seventy-two hours of unprotected sex. Some religious groups argued that the availability of the morning-after pill would encourage casual sexual behavior. On the other hand, Planned Parenthood representatives said the pill could prevent about half of the three million unintended pregnancies each year. In theory this would reduce American fertility. In May 2004 the FDA ruled against the pill's producers but allowed for additional evidence to be provided. It is most unlikely that a final ruling will be made during the 2004 election year.

Sperm count. In early 2004 the Aberdeen Fertility Centre in Northern Scotland issued the results of a survey of 7,500 men tracked from 1989 to 2002. Their average sperm count fell by 29 percent. There have been other such studies, but nothing definitive.

Age of marriage. In December 2003, data from the National Center for Health Statistics showed that the average age of marriage in America was 25.1 years—the highest ever, and up from 21.4 years in 1970. Similar trends have been at work around the world. The 25.1 is an average. For those at the upper end of the range, conception for women becomes more difficult. Some argue that the sharp decline in fertility only represents a delay in fertility, not a true precipitous fall. But the data does not bear it out.*

Money. It has been a general precept of demographic Transition Theory that as people get richer, they have fewer children. In recent times people have indeed been getting richer. As we shall see, the rate of climb has been fastest in the Less Developed Countries. On the other hand, that *New York Times* headline—". . . A Dip in Birthrates Defies Old Theories"—referred to the idea that in poor countries fertility was falling in advance of socio-economic progress. In either event, fertility falls.

Sexually transmitted diseases. STDs have been rising. Some of them can cause infertility, further lowering Total Fertility Rates.

---

*In 1967, after the end of the baby boom, 31 percent of Americans thought "four" was the "ideal number of children for a family to have," according to a Gallup Poll. In 2003 the comparable number was 9 percent.

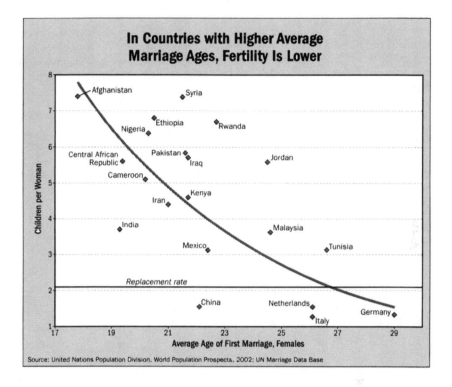

In Countries with Higher Average Marriage Ages, Fertility Is Lower

Source: United Nations Population Division, World Population Prospects, 2002; UN Marriage Data Base

Homosexuality. The emergence of the Gay Rights movement and the increasing acceptance of homosexuality would logically seem to lower fertility, albeit in quite small numbers. In earlier times when most homosexuality was kept "in the closet," some homosexuals would marry and have children. Now it seems that such a pattern would be less likely, with a consequent drop in fertility.

Cloning. In 1996 the cloned sheep "Dolly" was born in England. Since then there has been speculation that one day human beings too will be cloned, and that this might some day help solve the falling fertility problem. So far, no human clone has been produced. There have been medical problems with cloned animals. The potential problems for human clones would likely be monumental.

Until early in February 2004 it was assumed that no such research into human cloning was going on. Then a team of South Korean scientists published a paper in *Science* magazine providing a detailed description of how to create human embryos by cloning. The scientists declared that the purpose of their work was not to clone humans but to understand better the causes and treatment of disease, such as Parkinson's and diabetes. Anti-cloning advocates denounced the research.

In any event, even before the South Korean announcement most people found the idea distasteful. In autumn of 2002, Eurobarometer polled people in fifteen European countries, asking the yes-no question, "I would support the cloning of embryos to help infertile couples have children." The results showed 29 percent agreeing, 53 percent disagreeing, and 17 percent "don't know." In America in September 2003, a survey conducted by the Center for Public Policy, Virginia Commonwealth University, asked, "The technology now exists to clone or genetically alter animals. How much do you favor or oppose allowing the same thing to be done in humans—do you strongly favor, somewhat favor, somewhat oppose, or strongly oppose?" Thirteen percent strongly or somewhat favored; 84 percent were strongly or somewhat opposed.

"*Diffusion theory.*" Demographers and social scientists have begun to focus on the idea that cultural and economic changes of the sort iterated above do not alone provide a complete explanation of why fertility falls or stabilizes. Diffusion theorists ask about the mechanisms that change attitudes toward fertility, particularly in the LDCs. At root they are talking about the modern revolution in communications.

Diffusionists note that the vast expansion of modern communications has allowed governments and nongovernmental organizations to spread their message of family planning to a far wider swath of the population than before. Modern ideas about smaller family sizes are more easily disseminated, without having to use incentives or coercion. False rumors about the harmful effects of family planning can be struck down.

The exponential growth of the modern communications web has been a wonder to behold. Computers, e-mail, cell phones, expanded phone systems, fax machines, copiers, CDs, and VCRs only begin a long list. Probably the most important "new" aspect of modern communications is somewhat older but has now become nearly universal on the planet: television. Today there is scarcely a spot in the world where the great majority of people do not have access to television reception, be it cable, satellite, or old-fashioned over-the-air. In the most remote areas of the LDCs, a single television set may serve a whole village in a communal setting.

Access to television spurs modernism. The tube presents a good deal of horrendous and vulgar junk, but eye-opening material as well. At times the commercial messages tell more about the nature of the new world than the programs themselves. A key message of modern television concerns materialism. People see what their money could buy if they had more money. And they would have more money per person if their families were smaller.

An interesting question arises. If mass communication can effectively explain to people in the LDCs that too many children are too many, might not the same communication web be used to explain to modern countries in Europe and to the Japanese that too few children are also a major problem? For the moment, television programming aimed at young people seems to work the other way. It glorifies the life of single young people, of sex without children, of music that encourages such behavior, of high standards of materialism.

Perhaps such diffusion is already under way. In early 2004 the German newsweekly *Der Spiegel* ran a cover picture of a young baby hoisting sixteen old Germans on a barbell. The headline on the cover read "THE LAST GERMAN—ON THE WAY TO AN OLD PEOPLE'S REPUBLIC." Perhaps, sooner or later, Germans will realize that they must do something if Germany is to remain in recognizable form. The key question is "How?" I don't know the answer any better than anyone else.

"*Capitalism is the best contraceptive.*" I was a Reagan-appointed U.S. delegate to the 1984 UN Population Conference in Mexico City. It was a time when demographic alarmism and explosionism were near their peak.

Although the U.S. delegation had a few population alarmists on our team (including Paul Draper, Jr., then head of the Population Crisis Committee), the principal position of the U.S. government was both "conservative" and "moderate," depending on how one chose to look at it. The co-chairmen of our delegation were Alan Keyes and Senator James Buckley, and by anyone's standard they would both be called conservatives. In fact they would be insulted if they were not so designated. Yet their position was quite moderate, at least as I saw it.

An early draft of the U.S. position paper, prepared by lower-level hard-line mice at the National Security Council, caused great consternation when it was leaked. (What position paper coming from Washington isn't leaked, causing great consternation?) As I recall, the original draft became deeply enmeshed in an emotional disquisition of the abortion debate. I told the more sensible and senior people who put together the final draft position paper that I couldn't serve on the delegation if that was to be our position. Senior officials changed the language, and not because of me. The document emerged as what is still called the "Mexico City" position.

The general and most important thrust of the statement said, in effect: "Population growth, by itself, is a neutral phenomenon." That is, what's important is not how many people there are (within reasonable limits), or whether they are growing or diminishing, but how those people are behaving economically.

The alarmist case was something quite different, at least for the Less Developed Countries. The conventional wisdom of the time (and, to a lesser degree, now) was that a growing population meant more people sharing a common pie, reducing portions for all. The Reagan administration presented another view. The position paper explained that if the poor economies of the world paid more attention to the market principles of economics, rather than to bureaucratic socialism, they could prosper, just as the United States had prospered while its population was increasing at the fastest rate in human history.

The Mexico City meeting, like most UN international conclaves, was an enormous affair, including delegates from more than 150 countries, plus missions from many nongovernmental organizations, journalists, and hangers-on. Almost without exception, the gathering believed in the alarmist side of the debate. For them the Reagan position was a Neanderthal joke.

Their reaction was summed up by signs and campaign buttons prepared by some of the nongovernmental organizations that said "Capitalism Is the Best Contraceptive."

This was regarded as bizarre and heretical. I remember standing with Julian Simon outside the conference hall during a break in the proceedings. He was an emotional man, and he was disconsolate.

Don't any of them understand? Why won't they listen? His training was in economics and marketing, and he was particularly incensed that honored and historic economic views that went back at least to Adam Smith were not only ignored but mocked.

My own view was that the joke was on them. A pretty good case can be made that capitalism indeed may be the best contraceptive. Socialism may have taken men to the barricades, but countries practicing democratic capitalism have created far more wealth for their people than have those societies where socialism has been practiced. And wealth, as we have seen, typically correlates with low fertility.

Fertility enhancement. In the last few decades an entire industry of "fertility enhancement" has emerged. Many millions of people want to have children and cannot have them, a circumstance that often represents great human tragedy. Tune in your car radio to hear advertisements from "fertility clinics" or individual practitioners. Sometimes they promise success "or your money back."

A variety of fertility enhancement techniques are now being offered. At the most elemental is plain and sound education. Some patients need to know what days in a woman's menstrual cycle she is most fertile. Beyond that, according to the American Society for Reproductive Medicine (ASRM), it is astonishing what some Americans don't know. Obstetricians report that some (few) women have to be told that the natural way to go about reproduction requires intercourse. Some (few) women have to be told which is the proper orifice to use for reproduction.

But sophisticated artificial means of reproduction have produced heartwarming results. The ASRM, based on data from Centers for Disease Control, reports that about 1 percent of babies born in America are born through procedures "external to the womb," specifically in vitro fertilization ("test-tube babies") and intercytoplasmic sperm injection, a variant of in vitro.

Most fertility enhancement procedures are "internal to the womb." They include fertility drugs, artificial insemination, and hormone replacement. Reliable data for births through these means are not available, according to the ASRM, but it is surely likely to be higher than the 1 percent figure for "external to the womb" treatments. Again, the results can yield a set of extremely happy parents.

There are some downsides to fertility enhancement. About 40 percent each of internal and external procedures yield multiple births, typically twins and triplets. The "natural" rate of multiple births for women nearing the end of their childbearing years is about 20 percent, which is substantially higher than the rate for younger women. Multiple births (triplets and above) tend to yield babies that are somewhat more likely to have birth defects and medical problems, which would typically be apparent shortly after birth. (The principal cause of these problems would be premature birth and low birthweight.) Medical costs for these conditions can be quite high and are often not covered by medical insurance. Some procedures, such as "surrogate motherhood," can involve expensive legal fees. Some of the treatments can be painful to the woman.

With all the techniques, and all the joy brought to parents, the numbers involved are still sufficiently small that they have very little influence on the overall demographic numbers.

Cohabitation. When I was growing up, cohabitation was called "living in sin." Later the Census Bureau gave it an official name: "Persons of Opposite Sex Sharing Living Quarters," or "Posselque" in the demographic argot. It is quite common in America and so common in Europe that it is barely remarked upon. The general evidence indicates that posselques have fewer children than nonposselques, and that the unions are more likely to end than marital unions.

Sex ratios. When more female fetuses are aborted than males, it creates a future "bride shortage," lowering fertility.

Pro-natalism. Can something be done about low fertility? Should something be done about it? If so, the proper laboratory to look at would be Europe. The rubric is called "pro-natalism," and the European nations have worked hardest at it. Over the years many billions of francs, deutsche marks, pounds, and guilders have been put into major efforts for day care, maternal leave, paternal leave, flex time, children's allowances, housing allowances, mortgage preferences, and many more programs that smart social welfare legislators have proposed. (The United States does some of the same through its children's tax credit and other programs.)

Yet European TFRs have fallen dramatically. The argument can be made that rates would have fallen even lower without such pro-natal activity. Such programs may indeed be good on their own merits. But the fact of the matter is that pro-natalism as a means of seriously boosting fertility has not worked well.

A recent study of twenty-two industrialized nations from 1970 to 1990 showed that family allowances—that is, cash benefits—did indeed work, but only by a minuscule amount.* An increase of 25 percent in family allowances yielded an increase of a little more than .05 of a child. In other words, such an increase would change a TFR from about 1.30 children per woman to 1.35.

With all the inducements to raise European fertility, there remains the fact that European rates are the lowest in recorded history. Something isn't working.

Low and falling fertility is not a new problem in Europe, though the current hyper-low levels certainly are. In the 1930s, during the depression, the great French demographer Alfred Sauvy looked ahead gloomily and saw a continent of old people, in old houses, with old ideas. But the seminal work of the Swedish social scientist Gunnar Myrdal in helping to create the European welfare state was in large measure an attempt to provide an economic base so that young people could have children without worrying about how they would support themselves and their offspring.

Three cheers for pro-natal theory. But neither Europeans nor Americans now have that kind of money for the payout. Even with tax credits, the amounts of (pro-natal) monies going to children have been falling, in America and elsewhere. America once had a mildly serious pro-natal policy. Comedians used to josh a pregnant woman, "I see you're having a little deduction."

Could it be that we're not spending enough? In the late 1990s, C. Eugene Steuerle, an Urban Institute scholar and a tax official in the Reagan administration, made a calculation that put what was happening in perspective. Had the federal dependent tax exemption kept pace with income and inflation growth since 1948, it would have been worth $10,042 instead of what it was in the late 1990s, $2,550. (An "exemption" is worth less in tax savings than a "credit,"

*Anne Gauthier and Jan Hatzius, "Family Benefits and Fertility: An Econometric Analysis," *Population Studies* 51 (1997), 295–306.

but the $10,042 would have had a cash value of about $1,500 for a family in the 15 percent tax bracket and almost $3,000 in the 28 percent bracket.)

Some European demographers, Jean-Claude Chesnais of the Institut National Etudes Demographiques (INED) for one, thinks that has happened in Europe as well.

One big problem with pro-natal policies—even if they work, which the evidence does not bear out—is that they take a great deal of time. A baby born nine months from now won't even start paying into a national pension plans scheme for a generation, until that baby matures and begins working. And, of course, that happens only after the country puts out a lot of money to raise and educate the child.

In theory, set at proper levels, pro-natalist programs *must* work. Consider the current American plan of tax credits for children, a variant of the European family allowance. Until the Tax Bill of 2001, parents of children received a $500 check per child per year. It was then raised to $1,000 per child per year. Senator John Kerry has a plan to raise it even further, keyed to income. Well, one might say that $1,000 a year is not anywhere near enough to raise a child. True enough. How about $10,000 per year? Or a million dollars? Sooner or later it would work; too bad there is not that kind of money around, in America, in Europe, or anywhere else.

Most all European governments are queasy about asking their citizens to reproduce in greater numbers for the sake of national growth or survival. That would be regarded as overt nationalism, which is what Hitler preached.*

Adoption. In a way, adoption can be regarded as pro-natal. Consider a pregnant sixteen-year-old girl. Neither she nor her boyfriend wants to get married, or cohabit. If the girl kept the child, it would be difficult for her to pursue an independent career. She disapproves of abortion. The girl gives the child up for adoption, to a couple who have been unable to have children, making them deliriously happy. The girl completes high school, goes on to college, gets married, and

---

*Estonia, population 1.4 million people, with a TFR of 1.2, is now paying new mothers a full year's salary and claims that fertility will rise by 20 percent in the first year. Perhaps so. But will it constitute an acceleration of births that would have occurred later, or a permanent increase? We shall see.

bears a child. Net gain: one "extra" child, or more if the woman and her husband make a decision for a larger family. The problem with adoption is that in most places it is very difficult to find a child, and is often inordinately expensive.

IT IS CLEAR that there are more aspects of fertility pulling it downward than pushing it upward. Something is going on that gives every indication of continuing, with very little evidence of a turnaround. It is a strange time. Joe Chamie notes that in nations with below-replacement fertility, the polling regarding "ideal number of children" results are now closer to one than two, which is a remarkable change.

TOGETHER, many of these items contribute to what is called the Second Demographic Transition, a popular theory put forth by demographers D. J. van de Kaa and Ron Lesthaeghe in the late 1980s. It has been called by the European Association for Population Study "the mainstream concept among popular scholars dealing with demographic change in European societies." In a word it could be described as "modernism." It includes falling fertility, cohabitation, childbearing outside of marriage, less formal levels of marriage, divorce, sharing of housework, the new freedom of sexual behavior, and the urge toward self-realization. Those who accept the idea of the Second Demographic Transition believe it is irreversible and universal in developed societies. They have no idea about how to raise fertility. The demographer Steven Sindig, director general of the International Planned Parenthood Federation in London, says, "The question is not whether European states *can* boost their fertility. It's whether they want to."

Part Two

WHAT CAN HAPPEN

The course of human history can be seen as a balance between grand clear events and more disguised processes. The beginning of World War II, for one example, might best be seen as a crashing event, with enormous consequences. On the other hand, the advent of the Industrial Revolution is better understood as a process, not an event. It happened over the course of several hundreds of years and is still happening. The repercussions were enormous and continue to reverberate.

The coming of the New Demography is best seen as a process, not an event. When fertility rates shrink from 2.1 children per woman to 2.0 or 1.9, there is no sound of booming cannons. When total population declines by one-tenth of a child per year, we do not see planes catapulted from aircraft carriers. The proper analogy is more prosaic. Consider a savings bank account operating on reverse compound interest. During the first few years the losses are small. Then they pick up speed. Sooner or later you take what's left of your money out of that account or you won't have anything left.

For good or for ill, or for both, global birthrates and fertility rates are down and headed much lower. Couples will have many fewer children than before, and many fewer than had been expected. Accordingly, global population will peak at a level lower than predicted, and will begin to shrink, though the timing and amount of shrinking are subject to argument. I figure global population will not go much over 8 billion and then begin contracting. That is a far cry from the long-term 10 billion people that the UN was projecting for 2150 based on its 1998 projections, very far from the 11.5 billion of the UN projection just a decade ago, and wildly below the 15 to 20 billion forecasts that were in vogue a few decades ago.

From all indications, the depopulation to come will not be a short-term affair. Turning around a reverse geometric progression is not easy. "Demographic momentum" works on the downside just as it does on the upside: exponentially. Women, on average, must bear 2.1 children just to stay even over an extended period of time. But once that replacement rate has been substantially breached and remains below replacement over an extended period of time, as it already has in Europe and Japan, a different dynamic takes over. Previous population levels will not be restored even if the TFR returns to 2.1 children per woman (unless there is an implausible amount of immigration). After all, the new mothers would have to come from a thinned cohort. Four to five children per woman would be closer to the mark to reestablish previous population levels within a reasonable time frame.

If you believe that European or Japanese or American women will begin bearing an average of four children in the relatively near future (or Mexican, Iranian, and Brazilian women for that matter), you are reading the wrong book. Just consider that in America, private-college tuition in the better schools runs between $30,000 and $40,000 per year in after-tax money. Public-school college tuition is less but is going up almost everywhere and is cheap almost nowhere. Try putting four kids through college at those costs. If you have a masochistic streak, add in graduate school expenses. (Poor young Americans bent on getting advanced education can get it, but it may not be an easy matter.)

Nor is an apparent change in the works. Carl Haub, chief demographer at the Population Reference Bureau, tracks population statistics from all over the world and prepares annual extensive data charts. Says Haub: "As of April 2002 there has been no sign of increase." Most every demographer agrees with that view.

Of course, there are always small local stories of rates going up or down. The Swedes have crowed because fertility is up—by less than .1 child. A Canadian of Sri Lankan heritage is interviewed and tells why she and her second-generation friends are having fewer children than her first-generation immigrant parents. In 2004 the demographer Martin Vaesson at Measure DHS says Kenya's TFR is really 4.9, not the 4.0 that the UN reports, and seems to be stagnating. At the same time he says that Kenya is an exception and that most African nations have declining TFRs. The French have been expending considerable funds on pro-natal practices, and in the last quarter-century the French TFR soared from 1.86 children per woman to 1.89. (Some observers believe that a small part of the relatively high French TFR is attributable to its comparatively high population of Arab descent.) And there is the stunning drop in 2002 South Korean fertility described earlier.

What might all this mean?

CHAPTER EIGHT

The Graybe Boom

WE WILL SEE lower fertility rates and then falling population, likely for quite a while, engendering major changes. What will the effects of the New Demography be, salutary or sad?

Attempting to thoroughly explore the wide avenues and narrow alleys of possibility in such a situation would yield an encyclopedia, a large and incomplete one at that. There are no solid answers. Demography may offer better clues about the future than other social sciences, but they are clues, not certainties.

So I offer here some speculations based on the facts laid out in Part One of this book. I deal here with topics we hear a great deal about: pensions, commerce, the environment, geopolitics, and immigration. Many more topics could be added; they too would have to be dealt with speculatively. In any event, we will all be affected, personally, nationally, and internationally. The common theme of the New Demography—no surprise—is babies, or lack thereof.

We begin with the aging of the population and the problems it can cause.

IN THE FIRST PARAGRAPH of a publication of the European Commission,* the authors Kieran McMorrow and Werner Rogers write that the implications of aging populations ". . . will be significant in terms not only of a slowdown in the growth rate of output and

---

*"Economic and Financial Market Consequences of Ageing Populations" (2003).

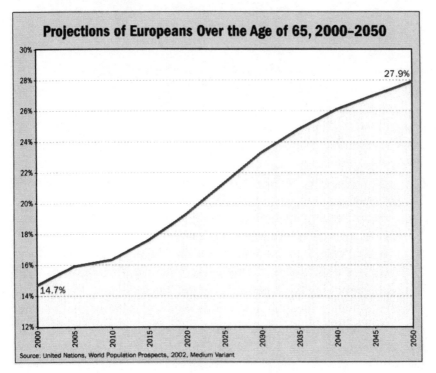

Projections of Europeans Over the Age of 65, 2000–2050

27.9%

14.7%

Source: United Nations, World Population Prospects, 2002, Medium Variant

living standards but also with regard to fiscal and financial market trends . . . falling rates of capital accumulation and a slowdown in productivity growth. . . . The coming decades bode *ominously* . . ." (my italics).

And the opening paragraph of the "2003 Aging Vulnerability Index" by Richard Jackson and Neil Howe, published by the Center for Strategic and International Studies (CSIS) and Watson Wyatt Worldwide, declares, "The rapid aging of the developed countries will pose a *major challenge* for global prosperity and stability during the first half of the twenty-first century" (my italics). Jackson says funds promised are so large they cannot be measured—and are at least in the *quadrillions* of dollars.

Indeed, the New Demography creates an imbalance between senior citizens and the rest of the population. So many old people! New medicines, better public sanitation, and behavioral changes have added years to life and often life to years. It is happening most everywhere in the world that is not blighted by the pandemic of HIV/AIDS or collapsing health delivery systems. That is the good news. But who will pay for the public pensions of the senior citizens if there are only comparatively few worker bees in the population? And who will pay for medical care for the seniors? After all the crisis-mongering about the situation, how serious is it?

There is an irony at work: a principal cause of the aging boom is a baby bust. The median age in America in 1950 was 30. By 2000 it was 35. In 2050 it is expected to be 40. In Europe in 1950 the median age of the population was 29 years. In 2000 it was 38 years. In 2050 it is projected to be 48. Japan had a median age of 22 in 1950, 41 in 2000, and an expected 53 in 2050.

Seen another way, in 1950 just 8 percent of Europe's population was over age 65. A hundred years later, in 2050, the projection is 28 percent.

But why are populations aging? Part of the received folk wisdom of our time is that the coming aging boom, with its attendant problems, is due to increased longevity. And indeed life expectancy has been extended dramatically. Life expectancy at birth for the entire world in the early part of the 1950s was 47 years; in 2000 it was 65 years, and in the UNPD projections it is slated to be 74 years in the latter years of the 2045–2050 time frame. The counterpart numbers for just the modern nations are 66 years, 76 years, and a projected 82 years. Amazing. And these numbers show the gain only from 1950; they don't even count the vast increase in life expectancy from 1900 to 1950. In America, for example, life expectancy at birth shot up from 49.5 years in 1900 to 69 years in 1950, to 77 in 2000, and a projected 82 in 2050. (Some medical researchers believe that life expectancy may climb substantially faster in the decades ahead. In April 2004 the New Jersey Medical School held a conference on aging and asked whether the average life expectancy might reach 120 by the year 2100. The UNPD projection for 2300 is a mere 95.)

The extension of life is remarkable, but it may seem like more than it is. The talk we hear is almost always about "life expectancy," but, as used above, that is just shorthand for "life expectancy at birth." A different picture emerges if a different demographic lens is used. Look at longevity at age 60 rather than at birth. In 1900, at the

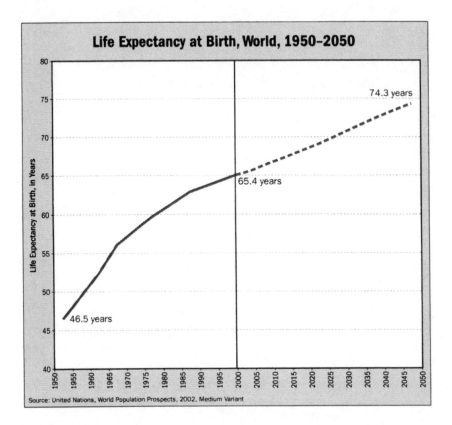

Life Expectancy at Birth, World, 1950–2050

74.3 years

65.4 years

46.5 years

Source: United Nations, World Population Prospects, 2002, Medium Variant

dawn of the twentieth century, a 60-year-old American could expect to live to age 75. By 2000, the end of that century, a 60-year-old American could expect to live to age 82, a seven-year increase, not the higher, double-digit numbers shown above. An extra seven years is nothing to sneeze at, but it is only one-fourth as long as the average increase of life expectancy of an American infant at birth living during the same time. The big demographic shifts come from fewer babies, not older adults.

Consider the data concerning the "median age" of the population. In the modern nations it was 29 years in 1950 and is projected to be 45 in 2050. Those numbers are heavily influenced by falling fertility. After all, the median is the middle number of an array of ranked numbers, and is moved by the quantities above and below the median. We live at an odd moment: a big baby boom followed by an unprecedented birth dearth. The median age, that is, the "person in the middle," is floating upward because so few young people are pulling it down. Meanwhile the flood of onetime babies of the Baby Boom is growing older, and closer to the retirement ages promised by governments.

In America the Baby Boom began in 1946, the year that both Bill Clinton and George W. Bush were born. Unless something untoward happens, they will have reached age fifty-eight by the time this book is published in 2004. But if the Boomers had matched their parents' fertility rates, or even split the difference between what was and what is, the American population would have a great many more younger people, pulling down what is now the projected median age and diminishing the cost problems of the pension and health-care situations. (If fertility rates fall gradually, public finance problems are diminished.)

So too with the data on "percentage aged." Had there been fatter cohorts in recent years, the percentage of people in their younger years would have increased. Instead American fertility has averaged 1.95 children per woman in the twenty-one years from 1981 to 2001.

These demographic trend lines will have a major economic impact on life in the twenty-first century. Many students of public finance are deeply concerned. Most state-run retirement programs in the modern countries, including America, are "pay as you go." That means that the government takes in money from currently working-age people and redistributes the same money to people who are currently of retirement age. Many countries operating under such a system proudly call themselves "welfare states."

In America, where "welfare" has become a bad political word, roughly the same sort of retirement plan is called "Social Security"—two golden political words. Conservatives, whose linear political ancestors condemned the system as a part of "creeping socialism," now swear to voters that they will do whatever is necessary to preserve and guarantee their cherished Social Security pension benefits.

Of course, in a pay-as-you-go system federal legislation could theoretically diminish those guaranteed benefits (called "entitlements") by raising taxes or raising retirement ages. Voters don't like either choice.

Many conservatives, dubious of government programs and policies, want people to own part of their pension plans—"partial privatization of Social Security." Conservative critics of Social Security call it a "Ponzi scheme" and claim it is made viable only by new young suckers joining the game to keep the cash flowing. In that sense Social Security is indeed a Ponzi scheme.

But all this is not new in history. Life itself is just such a scheme. In earlier times, aged and dependent parents were typically cared for by their working-age children, typically living within an extended family (and honored for their acquired wisdom and senior status). When those children themselves become aged or infirm, a new crop of children came along to care for them.

Nowadays a base of intergenerational care is accomplished through governments. The government systems have worked out rather well—so far. Not only have payments to the elderly been met, they have been expanded over the years. And in some respects Social Security works very well in human terms as well: senior recipients are less likely to feel "dependent" on their children. They get their money from Social Security (and they drive around in RVs with bumper stickers saying "We're spending our kid's inheritance").

In this pay-as-you-go system, money comes to seniors from taxes paid by their children and their employers in the form of Social Security payments. But no matter; after all, today's seniors put money into the system for their parents. Moreover, the benefit scale was regularly mandated upward until fairly recently, giving those already retired over age sixty a very good deal compared to people who will retire in the years to come. The trouble again comes when an unusually large cohort of people (Baby Boomers) produce an unusually small cohort of people (the birth dearth). The economist June O'Neill of Baruch College, former director of the Congressional Budget Office, calls it a "perfect storm." When the big cohort reaches its own age of retirement, the result is a shortfall of contributors to the pay-as-you-go plan. In America in 1955 there were nearly 9 workers for every retiree; today there are only 3.3. Under current projections, the ratio will fall to 2 workers for every retiree by 2035. Social Security payments will rise from 4.5 percent of GDP to 7 percent over the next three decades.

In Europe and Japan, with much lower TFRs, the numbers are even more daunting. This is the problem that has often been described as a looming crisis. The time of difficulties is fast approaching.

And it is just beginning. In 2000 there were 17 million people in the modern nations aged 85–99. The projection for 2050 is 62 million.

In America in 2002, Social Security medium projections showed "trust fund" surpluses of well over a trillion dollars to handle payouts. But as the Baby Boomers begin retiring around 2010, that "trust fund" will be drawn down each year. By 2017 it will be taking in less than it is scheduled to pay out. In the political lexicon of our time, that is often called "going bankrupt." And in 2041 the "trust fund" will be wholly exhausted.* At that time, if no changes are made in the current formula, retiring Americans would receive only about 70 to 75 percent of what they had been promised. This is called "going broke"—though if you or I go broke we would not usually continue to receive 70 to 75 percent of our income. Notwithstanding, it is a serious problem. (On the one hand, for many Americans, the "withholding" tax of Social Security is greater than their income tax. On the other hand, the contributor is actually buying a pension plan worth real cash.)

Note the quotation marks that have been placed around "trust fund." There is no trust fund. The Social Security money in question comes from general government revenues and is used to pay the regular costs of running a government, which have been rising under both Democratic and Republican administrations. To "save Social Security," politicians invent fictitious "lockboxes."

The alleged forthcoming American crisis will be mild compared to those of other modern countries. America still has a TFR near replacement; its retirement ages are somewhat older than in Europe and Japan; and we take in more immigrants, whose median age is twenty-eight and who will pay into Social Security for somewhat more than forty years before drawing benefits. Europeans generally retire earlier than Americans, in countries with desperately low TFRs, low immigration rates, and much older populations. (Examples of retirement age for men in 2000: Belgium, 58.1; France, 58.8; Germany,

---

*Some newer numbers push the year forward.

61.0; Italy, 59.7; Netherlands, 59.9; United Kingdom, 62.9; Sweden, 64.4; and Switzerland, 64.5.* The American retirement age was raised in 1983 to 67, which will take full effect by 2022.)

In the last few years, finally, politicians seem to be getting the message. But the voters are tough. In France in the summer of 2003, unions called strikes that tied up bridges, ports, train stations, airports, subway systems, and toll roads. But President Jacques Chirac's prime minister, Jean-Pierre Raffarin, did not back down on his plan to overhaul the French pension system. "This is about the survival of the republic," he told the French parliament. Similar strikes erupted in the same cause in many Western European nations. Italian unionists marched with signs that read "Defend Your Future." In March 2004 Chirac's center-right party lost power in most of France's regional assemblies. Election analysts ascribed the defeats to the government's policies on pensions and health care.

In 2004 the Austrian minister of education and science declared, "We are all living longer; there are fewer children. You can't strike against demographic developments like that."

And European/OECD nations are beginning to act. Germany, Canada, Sweden, and the United Kingdom have enacted policies to encourage fuller funding of their pension systems. Germany, Sweden, the UK, and the United States have enacted measures to reduce benefits. More will follow. They have to. The expenditures necessary to meet once-guaranteed pension costs are enormous and cannot be met without reduced benefits or increased taxes. Scotland's TFR is only 1.48, lower than the UK's 1.60. Some economists maintain that only if Scotland gets control of immigration from the UK will it be able to draw in young people to help pay the freight for pensions and trigger healthier economic growth.

A similar situation is in play in Southeast Asia. "Our falling birthrate is a cause of great concern" said Singapore Prime Minister Goh Chok Tong in a lunar New Year's message to his people. (The Singapore TFR was 1.36 children per woman in 2000–2005, compared to 4.93 children per woman forty years earlier in 1960–1965.) In 2000, Goh's government instituted a one-time "baby bonus," com-

---

*"Living Happily Ever After: The Economic Implications of Aging Societies" (2004), World Economic Forum developed with Watson Wyatt Worldwide. The data are for actual average age of retirement, not age of eligibility.

posed of subsidies, tax breaks, and other incentives, but so far it has failed to halt the fertility slide. Meanwhile the official family planning slogan for Singapore succinctly tells of the dramatic change in the fertility story in recent decades. It used to be "Stop at Two." Now it is "Three Children or More If You Can Afford It."

(The baby bonus package in Singapore did not impress a twenty-eight-year-old professional quoted by the *Daily Express News* in early 2004: "The baby bonus is only a one-off thing. I have two friends who just gave birth, and both are struggling." The quoted woman also announced that she might not have a baby until she was thirty-five.)

The innovative Singapore Ministry of Community Development and Sports has launched a government campaign designed to increase fertility by sponsoring two new perfumes, "floral" for women and "musky" for men, each called "Romancing Singapore Eau de Parfum." Keep your eye on the 2005 rates.

In Taiwan, government authorities are pushing for tax reductions and education subsidies to boost fertility rates.

In early 2004 the South Korean government proposed to raise the average retirement age from 57 to 60. Japan passed laws in 2003—a "Fundamental Law Against a Decline in the Fertility Rate" and "The Law to Support the Development of the Next Generation." We shall see. Pro-natalism does not have a good record. (But Singapore, Taiwan, and South Korea are low-fertility, relatively high-income Less Developed Countries. Not so with China. Economist Hu Angang of Quinghua University says that getting old before getting rich is China's big twenty-first-century problem: "We will have the social burden of a rich country and the income of a poor country. No country has faced the same circumstances before." Many of the other LDCs will face similar problems in the future, but will have an extra generation or so to try to cope with it.)

The political tendency is not officially unanimous. In 2004, Philippine President Gloria Arroyo told reporters that those countries that took vigorous family planning measures in earlier years are now facing low birthrates and consequent aging problems. Her policy abhors artificial contraception. Abortion is illegal. But she is fighting a losing battle. The TFR in the Philippines was 7.13 in 1955–1960; today it is projected at 3.18 and has fallen by one child per family in just ten years.

With all proposed changes, and with some new political courage, the pension problems are still far from being fixed. Stanford economist John Shoven says the root of the problem is "Europeanization." With the best of intentions, the European welfare states have reversed the incentives for work. They have generally promised relatively high pensions, in many cases linked to very early retirement ages, and with little loss of income for a person who retires. (Aside from the straight pension problem, Shoven maintains that such policies have played an important role in high taxation, which lowers the rewards for investment. He also believes that the Europeanization problem has afflicted America, albeit to a much lesser degree.)

As it happens, America has what seems to be one of the easier pension "fixes" available. The Cost of Living Adjustment (COLA) to Social Security is now raised each year according to an index based on wages, which have been rising quite rapidly over the years. A variety of plans have been suggested to change the index from "wages" to "prices"; it would be based on the Consumer Price Index (CPI), which rises more slowly than wages.

Such an index change could make a massive difference in the current projected Social Security shortfall, though it would require other changes in Social Security regulations. Under some of the plans, the *entire* shortfall would be eliminated. Of course, elected office holders of both parties, at least those who are seeking another term, have promised not to cut benefits. An index switch from wages to prices would indeed cut benefits. It could become a political football. On the other hand, it might be near invisible and avoid political fallout. Many low- and middle-income recipients could receive a higher real Social Security payment each month, just not as much as they would under the wages index.

FAR MORE SERIOUS than the pension situation are the circumstances of medical care. Pensions, like Social Security, are "capped." The government promises to pay a citizen a fixed amount of money, typically adjusted for inflation. As people live longer, costs may rise, but the promised pension payment in theory remains the same. With medical care, however, there is no cap. Scores of trillions of dollars are at stake.

A sixty-five-year-old goes into the hospital for a hip replacement. It is paid for by medical insurance. Two years later he or she has a mild heart attack. It is paid for by medical insurance. Two years later the covered individual—still working, by the way—is found to have cancer. The doctors say they caught everything in time, but the patient is asked to return to the hospital every six months for a thorough (and expensive) checkup. And so it goes. The covered individual takes good care of himself, lives for twenty more years, but spends the last months of life on life-support systems.

And that doesn't include insurance for prescription drugs, which until 2003 were not covered by federal insurance. Americans don't mount general protest strikes (not yet), but the politicians still act in ways that make existing problems more difficult, albeit for quite humanitarian reasons. When Medicare was established in 1965, the practice of medicine was quite different. For one, there were many fewer useful drugs on the market. So a drug benefit was not included. But many new and very useful medications have since become available, typically at high prices, sometimes at very high prices.

Senior citizens with no large savings or pensions often find drug prices unbelievably high. We see legitimately tragic television footage of poor old people saying they can choose either to eat or to pay for their drugs. ("Senior discounts" are available, but they don't discount very much.) The drug companies maintain, with merit, that they must make a profit to cover their huge costs of research, which include unsuccessful drugs that never make it to market. Otherwise, the companies say, fewer new drugs will be produced. (Estimates run to half a billion dollars in research costs per successful drug, and sometimes more.)

Both conservative Republicans and liberal Democrats opposed the presciption drug bill. Republicans said it cost too much and there wasn't enough money; Democrats said it was a cheapskate bill and the payout ought to be larger. There will always be politics.

Medical economist Joseph Antos of the American Enterprise Institute says the politicians are essentially ignoring the projected soaring costs of medical care. He believes that the political imperative that drove the prescription drug bill demonstrates that elected officials are (as ever) more interested in spending than saving. Indeed, the Medicare Trustees report of 2004 talks of a long-term shortfall of $8 trillion over the next seventy-five years. (Trillions sound cheap compared to the quadrillions mentioned earlier.)

Like pension benefits, health care has achieved the legislative status of "entitlement," as opposed to ordinary "discretionary spending" which is appropriated year by year. An entitlement is automatic; it is paid out without a specific congressional appropriation. It is regarded as much harder to change than normal spending. And because the end recipients of entitlements are not only the covered individuals but doctors, nurses, hospitals, and insurance companies (to begin a lengthy list), the beneficiaries of entitlements are typically well-to-do and well organized, able to exert great influence on legislators. Sooner or later (undoubtedly later), attention will be paid and the monies for medical costs will be found, mostly in the taxpayer's pocket.

Is there a solution to the health-care situation? For many years health-care theoreticians have maintained that there are great inefficiencies in the health-care system everywhere, but especially so in America, which spends a much higher proportion of its GDP on health care than do the Europeans. Do American doctors order too many tests? Are there too many referrals to specialists? Perhaps so. But health care is a very special kind of spending. When your child is sick, you want the very best care, and damn the expense. The theoreticians may be right, but that doesn't make it easier to solve the problem politically or personally.

And a huge proportion of health-care spending goes for the very end of life. A patient may run up enormous bills in and out of hospitals and in and out of long-term health care, residentially or institutionally. Theoreticians have noted this, and some have even raised the possibility of cutting off all or part of governmental health care when a patient is facing a serious terminal condition.

Growing old can be grim. On the other hand, Henry Aaron of the Brookings Institution, co-editor of *Coping with Methuselah*,* speculates whether increased life expectancy will yield years of physical vigor and mental alertness or years of physical debility and mental decline. He believes that recent trends indicate that, on balance, we may be lucky on this one.

Talk about difficult politics. It's one thing if an elderly parent tells his children to "pull the plug" if he or she is in a vegetative state or

*Brookings Institution Press, 2004.

kept barely alive by a variety of tubes. But for a politician to tell the ailing parent, or the middle-aged son or daughter who listens and votes, "You've had it, Mom. You're on your own, good luck. . . ." It is not likely to happen.

Finally, despite all the new medicines, new medical knowledge, fine doctors, new procedures, dedicated health-care personnel— everyone dies, except typically later than they used to. Those extra years of life will almost surely produce greater medical costs.

The 2002 report of the Center for Strategic and International Studies, "Meeting the Challenge of Global Aging," is a gloomy one. Unless we inaugurate a system of reform in the modern nations— now—the bank will be broken. We will see shrinking labor forces, a decline in savings rates which can diminish investment levels, and on and on. Still, my own view is that pension and health-care problems may be overstated, for a number of reasons.

People indeed will be living longer lives (assuming the projections hold up). If people live longer, it is no sin to change the rules and have them work longer in order to accumulate full retirement credits. Live longer, work longer. Alas, most people, and most voters, don't seem to want to work longer.

Japan has one of the most serious aging problems in the world. Its post–World War II baby boom ended early; by the late 1950s the Japanese TFR was already below replacement, and sinking. (The French, English, and Germans didn't fall below replacement until the 1970s.) Today the Japanese TFR is at 1.3 children per woman, near the bottom of the array of nations, and with a very high life expectancy rate of 82, projected to climb to 88 in 2050.

Japan's is a classic pension crisis. The legal age of retirement there is age 59. If life expectancy indeed reaches 88 in 2050, that is 29 more years that the government must pay out pensions and health care. How can a nation possibly meet such commitments to its elderly? There will not be sufficient money coming in to pay for the actuarially determined number of years of retirement. In Tokyo a few years ago I asked that question of a Japanese demographer who had a simple answer: "Redefine 'aged,'" he said. "Pay pensions when people reach 70, not 60." Of course, demographers don't have to run for office. If Japanese politicians are like other politicians around the world, they will put off changing the rules almost until they are forced to, notwithstanding a somewhat more realistic attitude in recent years. The problem is as much political as gerontological.

In another way the pension problem is political rather than economic. While the median age of the population increases and more people are over age sixty-five, there will be proportionately fewer children. Children also draw on government monies. The "dependency ratio" (the proportion of persons over sixty-five added to those under fifteen in relation to those in their working years) will stay about the same as the decades move on. In theory the proportion of government funds now directed to the education of young people could be redirected to help the elderly. That is the theory. In practice it means a politician must vote to cut education expenditures or limit their rise. That is regarded as semi-suicidal politics.

Yet it may not be quite as politically difficult as imagined. In America it had been said that proposing changes in Social Security was like "touching the third rail" of politics. Yet in 1982 President Reagan set up a bipartisan commission to make recommendations for meeting the "going broke" crisis. Chaired by Alan Greenspan, with Senators Robert Dole and the late Daniel Patrick Moynihan as key elected players, the members agreed to a plan that extended the age at which Social Security would be available while gently raising taxes over time.

Congress passed the proposal; President Reagan signed it in 1983. There was no odor of singed flesh from the third rail. Reagan was elected by a landslide two years later. One key to success was that the rise in the age of eligible retirement was not to take place in 1983 but well into the future, and in tiny increments—hard to complain about. The third railers predicted that the sparks would begin flying when people found out that they could no longer get full retirement benefits at age 65. But under the phase-in approach, the age of retirement was not lifted until 2000, seventeen years into the future, and then rising only from age 65 to age 65 and 2 months. (Who will lead demonstrations against a two-month extension of the pension age?) Ultimately, under the 1983 reforms, the age of retirement would reach 67 by the year 2022. There have still been no political electrocutions.

Moreover, some disincentives to work have been removed from the system. It used to be that if an American continued working past age 65, he or she would likely receive no Social Security benefits until age 72, even among healthy people still willing and often anxious to work. This tended to encourage retirement as well as reduce production and Social Security revenues. In 2000 that restriction was repealed. Today Americans over the retirement age who continue to work receive full Social Security payments. I am one such person, delighted to receive the payments. But I have put in a good deal of money over the course of about fifty years in the work force. While I'm working, and while I'm receiving benefits, I'm still paying into Social Security. That helps keep the Ponzi scheme alive and running. (The Progressive Policy Institute has proposed a "Boomer Corps," to provide a tax-free $400 per month income to recent retirees who work at least 25 hours a week in civic projects, plus a $4,000 education voucher. It sounds like a policy idea headed in the right direction.)

Further, we should remember that when Social Security was established in 1935 it was regarded as only one leg of a three-legged stool. In the ideal vision, workers would also have personal savings and a company pension. Indeed, most Americans have at least some assets other than Social Security. At age sixty-five in 2000, Social Security payments provided for all the income of just 20 percent of elderly Americans. The rest have some personal savings or company or union pensions to augment their Social Security benefits. (Today Social Security payments range from $572 per month to $2,045 per month, a very long way from wealth even at the higher levels.)

We should not blame the architects of Social Security. Back in 1935, the average person died before receiving any benefits. Still, too many elderly Americans are not receiving enough money for a dignified retirement (though median income for those over sixty-five is now somewhat higher than the all-American average).

Help is on the way. Ever-greater numbers of Americans are investing part of their paychecks in government-sanctioned private retirement plans—IRAs, Keoghs, Roths, 401-Ks. Because they convey tax advantages, these plans are encouraging people to save privately for their own future. According to the Federal Reserve, 52 percent of American families had investment holdings in 2001, up from 32 percent in 1989, and 19 percent in 1983. Critics say that many investors have only small amounts in those plans. True enough. But the economist Eric Engen of the American Enterprise Institute calculates that in a 401-K plan, if a young man age 25, earning $40,000 a year, stays with the program he should end up with about $1.16 million by age 65. Engen's criteria include 6 percent of salary as employee contribution, employer match of 50 cents per dollar, annual growth in wages of 4 percent, return on stocks of 8 percent and bonds 4 percent.

In the wind are plans to "partially privatize" Social Security. In 2000, George W. Bush ran for the presidency on a platform that included a pledge to convene a commission to make recommendations to partially privatize Social Security. Bush was not electrocuted; he was elected.

The commission was appointed, co-chaired again by Senator Moynihan, and made its report in 2001. Three different plans for partial privatization were presented, with none singled out as the best. When the stock market "bubble" burst, the political momentum behind any privatization plan disappeared. But in 2003 and 2004, as the stock market recovered, President Bush promised to put it back on the front burner for the 2004 presidential campaign.

I believe the partial privatization of Social Security makes great sense. Yet, among the most adamant opponents of the plan is the AFL-CIO. I find it hard to imagine that the legendary labor leader Samuel Gompers, whose slogan was "More," would oppose the plan. After all, partial privatization allows workers to grow their wealth just as rich folks do, by investment.

The most publicized of the various plans now in play calls for allowing young and middle-aged workers to choose voluntarily to invest up to 3 percentage points of the 12.5 percentage points that currently come from the worker's and employer's donations to Social Security. Some partial privatization plans go as high as 6 percent input by those enrolled in Social Security (which is most everyone). Under such plans, Social Security would remain as it is for persons currently over age fifty. For younger people, the monies would go into a personal account that could be invested in a wide variety of financial instruments, including stocks, bonds, or money market funds.

The attack on partially privatized Social Security has centered on the notion that the assets in individual accounts would be put at severe risk in the event of a drop in the stock market. But that scenario is dubious. Jeremy Siegel of the University of Pennsylvania has investigated the behavior of the New York Stock Exchange going back to its inception in 1792. In his 1994 book *Stocks for the Long Run*, he observes that in 210 years there has not been a single instance that the value of NYSE stocks, counting dividends, has fallen over a ten-year span. That includes the years of the Great Depression in the 1930s.

The average annual return on stocks over the years has been 7 percent, after discounting for inflation. By contrast, the current Social Security system returns about 1 percent for young workers. The comparison is not exact by any means. Social Security payments also fund disability insurance and provide life insurance benefits for minor children if the breadwinner dies or is disabled. Those are very important benefits. Still, the difference in rewards between a partially privatized system based on investment and a government one running on a pay-as-you-go basis is quite substantial.

And should the unprecedented happen, should markets go into a truly long swoon, the government can provide for a protective cushion to make up a substantial portion of the differential—say 70 to 75 percent—in which case the argument for recipients getting hurt by a "risky scheme," as it has been called, would be much diminished. (And it would provide good Keynesian spending in a time of economic difficulty.)

Partial privatization is a good idea. It has already been adopted in England, Chile, Australia, Brazil—all told about twenty countries so far, and the number is growing. Sooner or later, given our demographic circumstances, some form of privatization plan is almost a certainty, in America and in most other modern countries. Partial privatization would be a key victory of capitalism, or, if you prefer, socialism. In either event, just plain people end up owning an ever-greater share of the means of production.

But partial privatization can do more. There is a difference between guaranteed wealth and guaranteed income. The latter, like Social Security, ends when the recipient dies. The former provides an estate that can be bequeathed to children, to charities, to whomever and whatever the owner decrees. In theory, if they meet certain financial standards to cover their retirement, recipients might be able to borrow against their private accounts while they are alive, much along the model of a home equity loan.

Finally, and perhaps most important, the partial privatization of Social Security could set in motion a small political and psychological revolution. It would provide most every young and middle-aged American a share of the American economy ("a piece of the Rock" in the old Prudential Insurance slogan). As the years go on and the current codgers move on to their reward, every adult American would own a share of the American economy. That might well diminish the class warfare "us versus them" mentality that too often scars American politics, and politics everywhere. We and the other democracies would do well to diminish such sour politics.

The modern nations have indeed dug themselves into a hole of public financing from which it will be difficult (but not impossible) to emerge. The critics of political profligacy say of the gutless politicians, "They're mortgaging our children's future."

Well, yes. But these same spendthrift politicians, or their earlier counterparts on both sides of the Atlantic, put up many trillions of dollars to do some very important things for posterity. One is defense spending. Were it not for such massive spending, the chances that the Soviet Union would have established a Communist presence in Western Europe cannot be dismissed. At the least, Western Europe might have become "Finlandized," that is, left alone but told to be quiet and not to make trouble.

IT HAS BEEN SAID that the essence of human wisdom is to have your cake and eat it too. Aging and its attendant problems are surely serious. We have, however, several factors operating in our favor. Thanks to remarkable technological and scientific progress, economic productivity (production per worker) has surged, albeit with plenty of bumps in the road. If the future resembles the past, economic productivity will continue to climb and people will be privately richer than they are now, even if their governmentally funded benefits are diminished. Indeed, people most everywhere are richer now than at any time in history. (After adjusting for inflation, median income for Americans grew from $13,148 in 1960 to $32,646 in 2000, as calculated in constant 1996 dollars. European incomes too have soared in the post–World War II years, though the last few years have been less than stellar.)

What workers may lose in pension and health benefits they may gain by growing richer in the private sector, paying for their own needs. Indeed, they may well come out ahead. Remember that the basic idea is to provide for the citizens, not balance the books.

If because of demographic imbalances or other economic reasons we cannot foresee, the economic growth we have witnessed for several hundred years slows down, it is nevertheless likely to be a problem of people growing richer at a somewhat slower pace. That has happened before, and we humans have survived pretty well.

As for Social Security, senior Americans will receive at least the major portion of their payments. They paid in, they should get their money out when they retire. But they are not really getting *their* money out of the system. Remember, this is a pay-as-you-go system. They are getting their money from currently working-age people.

Now, suppose Mr. and Mrs. Jones decided never to have children. Are they "free riders" when they reach retirement age? They will get their pension money from the children of Mr. and Mrs. Smith, who had three. Is that fair? The Joneses avoided the costs of raising children; they could have built up a major nest egg for retirement. Smith, on the other hand, paid to raise his kids and send them to college. He and Mrs. Smith had difficulty saving for retirement.

Suppose it were legislated that only *parents* received Social Security payments upon retirement. Such a harsh remedy will not happen, and shouldn't. Besides, there are too many voters without children. But some formula for recipients that accounted for the number of births might be worth thinking about.*

Finally, let us reemphasize that the pension and health circumstances are triggered in large part by very low fertility. We can speculate about future outcomes with good math and smart analysts, but we really don't know how it will all play out. The situation has not occurred before. It is a part of the New Demography.

*Former Japanese Prime Minister Yoshiro Mori said in 2003 that "The government takes care of women who have given birth to a lot of children as a way to thank them for their hard work. . . . It is wrong for women who haven't had a single child to ask for taxpayer money . . . after having enjoyed their freedom and fun."

CHAPTER NINE

Business

AN AGING POPULATION comes about in large measure because birthrates are down. When birthrates sink low enough, and stay low, countries eventually lose population. As we have seen, put together in their current global configurations, these situations can cause economic turmoil of the first magnitude in the developed modern world. We have seen it through the lens of aging and the public burdens it puts on governments. Now let us look at it through the lens of commerce.

The New Demography will play a major role in the economy of the next few decades, both positive and negative. The steep decline of fertility will likely yield commercial problems in the modern nations (America excepted). At the same time there is a window of great opportunity for real and substantial economic growth in the Less Developed Countries. It may well be of great importance to forward-looking businessmen and the world economy at large.

Various lists over the years have showed what industries get helped and what industries get hurt as population shifts occur in modern economies. For example, cruise lines, cardiology, geriatric care, reverse mortgages, health care, and cemeteries receive a boost from an aging population. On the other hand, orthodontists and youth clothing retailers lose out. But, at essence, these are switch-jobs: the orthodontist becomes a geriatrician. One job lost, one job gained.

On the downside, however, consider real estate. It involves more than simple job-switching. A growing domestic population demands additional housing. So builders build, carpet makers make carpets, furniture makers make furniture, and so on. There is a demand, too, for additional office space. Tall buildings rise. Desk makers manufacture desks. Computer makers, and those who make routers and servers, all feel demand and respond to it, creating jobs and profits, both in America and in foreign lands. Doctors examine patients. Automobile mechanics fix cars. Domestic workers find it easier to get jobs. A growing population in a modern country with sound policies tends to spur economic growth; it creates demand.

(Periodically, to be sure, the play of the free market yields economic turmoil. But since the 1930s in the United States, recessions have generally been comparatively brief or shallow, or both. This is in quite remarkable contrast to earlier American history where major economic swings—booms and busts—were somewhat commonplace. The same has been true in Europe.)

In real estate it is somewhat different when population is more or less stable. There are some teardowns, some new buildings and renovations going on, both residential and business. Some people buy second homes or time-share condos. Doctors still have patients. Cars get older and have to be repaired or replaced. This sort of steady-state economy should be able to do rather well. Economic productivity—"productivity" is the magic word in growth economics—per worker can increase, and everyone can live happily ever after.

From 1990 to 2000 the population of Europe grew from 722 million to 728 million, about stable. For many years European economies flourished; more recently they have grown more slowly, but still there has been growth and certainly no economic catastrophe. Real productivity growth can create a higher standard of living even as population remains stable.

But what happens when populations shrink? Continent-wide, Europe is projected to begin its decline in 2000–2005—now—with a small 653,000 person decline each year, a mere .09 percent. But the decline grows larger, reaching an annual drop of 3 million a year by 2050.

The fact is that we don't really know what happens to an economy in a sharply shrinking demographic situation. Since the advent of modern economics, going back at least to the beginnings of the

Industrial Revolution, there is no model for it. That should be emphasized and reemphasized.

But if you have an MBA, or you are a plain old modern entrepreneur, or a buyout specialist, these days you must have a model. So a question arises: Why would a businessman invest stockholder money in companies that depend in part on domestic sales when domestic markets are growing smaller and smaller? Perhaps I exaggerate, but this is a potentially quite serious situation—putatively profit-making businesses marching off into the unknown. (Economist John Shoven agrees that vacant real estate and declining populations may well be the canaries in the coal mine. Empty dwellings can have a depressing effect on the labor force and on new capital formation. In turn, this yields a lower rate of return, empty factories, and fewer customers.)

For at least several hundred years the population of Europe has done nothing but grow, even as the continent exported immigrants to the United States and elsewhere. In America, a high-fertility nation with high immigration rates and wide-open spaces, the growth has been near incredible. The first U.S. Census in 1790 enumerated somewhat under 4 million people, about the population of Greater Atlanta today. By 2005 the nation will have grown 75-fold, to about 300 million people. By 2050 the Medium Variant projection calls for 400 million. Later we shall ask whether such growth is good for America and for the world.

What we know is that we have had vast economic growth in the modern world and vast population growth—simultaneously. No one knows how tightly these variables are linked, but it would appear that there is at least some linkage. We had a customer boom. We had a wealth boom. What we have had has been good.

But how will nations react to what we have never had, a serious ongoing population decline, a customer dearth? Losing 100 million Europeans—or more—in the next 50 years will take us into economic terra incognita. Going from known and successful dry land to an unknown place makes economists think about phrases like "forthcoming crisis."

Of course, it's never easy to run a successful business in a highly competitive economy, but it is much easier to do so when the population is growing. Recall the front covers of the great American business magazines—*Business Week, Forbes, Fortune*—before the dot.com bubble burst. There was smiling Jack Jones. The cover line read "Jones Grows Acme Industrial." Sales were up at Acme, revenues and profits were up at Acme, and there seemed to be no end in sight. Jones was a remarkable businessman—so shrewd, such a visionary.

Well, yes. As the 76 million Baby Boomers went from infancy to middle age, as the American population grew by 130 million people from 1950 to 2000, there was one thing Jack Jones had going for him: a customer boom. If widgets were your game, there were 130 million new customers for widgets. Acme would make them. True, your wily competitors might gain a good share of new widget buyers, but there was a margin for error. Jack Jones and his chroniclers seemed to regard him as a man who could call up a mighty commercial wave for the greater glory of Acme Industrial. Without disparaging Jack's business skills, he and his fellow CEOs were like economic ships riding high on a mighty demographic wave and congratulating themselves for their power to call up the high surf.

But what's going to happen to Jack Jones's European counterpart, Heinz Hoerst, and his employees, and the European economy in which he participates, when the number of customers shrinks, substantially? Consider real estate again. Over a period of decades in Europe there will be fewer buyers for existing properties. Less demand for a constant supply yields lower prices. Lower prices yield lower values upon which to finance loans to provide for investment capital, diminishing both jobs and profits. (On the other hand, buyers will find lower prices for real estate.)

Not only that, but many of the furniture makers, carpet makers, and auto mechanics will find themselves with shrinking sales, revenues, and profits. There will be fewer jobs, but fewer people who need jobs. That may turn out to be a wash, though perhaps in a demoralized country. Herr Hoerst may find himself on the cover of a business magazine, but the story may well be about how he led his company into the pits.

I chose real estate as a prime example because, seen broadly, it may well be the largest industry in the world—from dishes to paint to wood, to begin a very long list. It's a volatile market in any event. Many economic observers believe that the long Japanese economic troubles were triggered by the popping of the Japanese real estate bubble. And, perhaps not coincidentally, that happened when Japanese demographic growth had just about ceased. Japanese population rose just 3 percent from 1990 to 2000, despite a TFR below 1.5 (the effect of demographic momentum). Japanese population was projected to plateau shortly after 2010 and then begin falling by a large number to the middle of the century and beyond. There weren't many new buyers clamoring to buy those overpriced Japanese office buildings and apartments, at least not at the old prices.

Now, all this is not set in concrete. Many economic thinkers are trying to figure out ways to deal with the New Demography. A large two-year study by the Center for Strategic and International Studies, "Meeting the Challenge of Global Aging," was chaired by Walter Mondale, Ryutaro Hashimoto, and Karl Otto Pöhl. The study lists thirty-three separate recommendations, some of which have as many as five subcategories, and thirty "findings," some with "subfindings." These are filled with "significant challenges," "underestimating consequences," and "serious risks." It is not a happy document.

But the study has ideas: More exports and more international out-sourcing can help a depopulating country. More deregulation can boost productivity. Replace pay-as-you-go pensions with privatized and funded pensions. Encourage people to work longer before retirement. Remove obstacles to pension portability. Prohibit age discrimination in the workplace. Restrain the use of mandatory retirement. End gender discrimination in the workplace. Encourage immigration. Promote tolerance among immigrant groups and natives. Promote tax reductions for parents with children and tax incentives for providers of child services. And, of course, hold more conferences.

Still, the CSIS study does not directly emphasize increasing fertility rates. Apparently the panel felt that any such course would be too late and too little. We have seen that pro-natal policies don't appear to do much good, and in any event the lag time until newly born infants finish a serious education and become serious producers and taxpayers is more than two decades, hardly a quick fix.

The commerce of the modern nations may slip the trap of the New Demography, but we should not delude ourselves: the trap is there, and it may well be serious.

IN RECENT DECADES we have thought of major economic growth as a feature of modern nations. Europe, America, and Japan have been the biggest players.

As this is written the American economy is doing quite well, growing at a rate of about 4.9 percent for the twelve months from the second quarter of 2003 through the first quarter of 2004, one full year (always subject to future change without notice). The recession of 2001 was brief but new jobs were slow in coming, and some called it a "jobless recovery"—particularly Democrats running for office. The Dow Jones and Standard and Poor's market indexes recovered much of their losses, though it will likely be a very long time before the NASDAQ high of 5,048 (March 10, 2000) is seen again. (On December 31, 2003, the NASDAQ closed at 2,003.) In some sense, it is remarkable that the U.S. and world markets have not experienced worse. After all, following the dot.com bubble came the explosions of 9/11, wars in Afghanistan and Iraq, and medical scares like SARS, Mad Cow disease, and avian flu.

The European economies have not done well in the past few years, perhaps for demographic reasons, perhaps not. The growth rate for the fifteen European Union nations for calendar year 2003 was 0.7 percent. Over the past five years (1999–2003) the EU growth rate was 1.9 percent. The comparable five-year U.S. rate was 2.8 percent.

Some gloomy economists look through the demographic lens and see the aging modern populations and their attendant costs. They see nations running out of assets to pay off their social commitments; they see voters unwilling to surrender benefits they feel they have earned. They look at the coming undersized fruit of the birth dearth. They wonder from where the next economic spur to growth will come from. Some commercial economists note that "major leaps forward" are rare occurrences in any event, and that even the 1990s may not have qualified.* In short, there are those within the economics community who are not optimists.

Now, this is not unusual. Within the economics community there are always long-term and short-term bulls and bears. Economists

---

*So wrote Sylvester J. Schieber (Wilson Wyatt Worldwide) for the Center for Strategic and International Studies, 2002.

have been said to predict seven of the last three recessions. It is called the dismal science.

But where might a "locomotive economy" be found to boost the global marketplace in the decades to come? A growing America might surely be one such place. But where else? It could come from Europe and Japan, as it has in the past, but I am dubious about finding locomotive wheels in countries that are losing stark numbers of customers and producers. There are, however, other exciting possibilities.

A 2003 report by the Rand Corporation entitled "The Demographic Dividend"* looks at the Less Developed Countries and comes up with a fairly optimistic view of the economic future. The authors review the arguments about the effects of population growth. "Pessimists" have maintained that rapid demographic growth is harmful because so many children require so many costly services, such as education, which inhibits the spending of resources for economically productive uses with a faster payoff. Over the years the pessimists have argued that only crisis-styled global family planning can save the situation.

Family planning is good in its own right. But the "optimists" have maintained that more people produce larger markets, an economy of scale, and more economic growth. They note that in the last thirty years population has doubled but per capita incomes have nonetheless increased by two-thirds.

Today, according to the Rand authors, it is the economic "neutralists" who have come to dominate the policy environment. The neutralists hold that nations can succeed or fail with high, low, or medium population growth. It's not how many people there are, it's what they do and how well they do it.

In this time of the New Demography, when fertility rates have already fallen dramatically in the modern nations and are now falling rapidly in the LDCs, broad new and healthy economic possibilities are plausible. The key to it, the Rand authors stress, is age structure.

Those searching for healthy ongoing growth should look at the Less Developed Countries. And within the LDCs the principal focus

* "The Demographic Dividend—A New Perspective on the Economic Consequences of Population Change" by David E. Bloom, David Canning, and Jaypee Sevilla (Rand Corporation, 2002).

must be on Asia, and within Asia on the two billionaire countries, China and India. More than 60 percent of the world's population is in Asia. And of that 60 percent, almost two-thirds are to be found in India and China. Both nations have seen enormous drops in TFRs. China's (now officially at 1.8 children per woman but probably somewhat lower) was achieved in part by coercive means, described earlier, and seems to have leveled off. The decline in India's TFR has been less dramatic, but a drop from 6 children per women (1950) to 3 children per woman today is nonetheless enormous. Some Indian states are already below replacement level.

This situation can yield the "demographic dividend." As fertility falls rapidly, as it is now doing in the LDCs, the national and personal costs of feeding, clothing, and educating children go down. It costs a family less to provide for a two- or three-child family than it did to provide for a much larger family in an earlier time. And there are positive ancillary economic effects. Once the youngest child reaches school age, for example, it is easier for women to find work in the money economy, thereby boosting national and personal income.

Most important, these children grow older. And even though they come from the relatively small families of the New Demography, there are hundreds of millions of them now, with more on the way in the years to come. Remember, their mothers were born a generation ago, before TFRs fell so low in the LDCs. Accordingly, a huge new young adult cohort is forming with unique characteristics.

They come from comparatively small LDC families. Their own families are projected to be smaller still. They are more likely to be educated, more likely to have access to family planning, more likely to live in a city than on a farm. Collectively they make up a huge and unique labor force in societies with less of a burden of child-related expenses, and with the consequent opportunity to create and save wealth, which produces jobs.

Well, you may say, that's all fine and good, but what about the already astronomically high unemployment rates one reads about in some of the LDCs—20 percent, 40 percent, or higher. Such numbers are grimly unfortunate, but they should be viewed in perspective. An "unemployed" man is not a starving man. We know that life

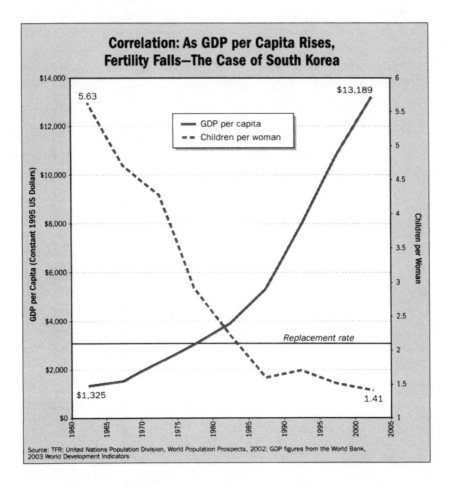

Correlation: As GDP per Capita Rises, Fertility Falls—The Case of South Korea

Source: TFR: United Nations Population Division, World Population Prospects, 2002; GDP figures from the World Bank, 2003 World Development Indicators

expectancy has gone way up in these countries, that caloric intake and physical size have increased. "Underemployment" or "insufficient employment," on or off the books, may be a better way to characterize much of what is called "unemployment."

As the Rand authors point out, an analogous situation occurred in East Asia during the quarter-century from 1965 to 1990. In those countries, fertility fell rapidly. In South Korea, for example, the TFR plunged from 4.7 to 1.7. During that time real per capita income growth grew by 6 percent per year, a powerhouse performance. And the demographic dividend—lots of workers with fewer dependents—accounted for 25 percent to 40 percent of economic growth, according to the Rand study.

Demography can give economic destiny a nudge, but no more than that. For the LDCs to capitalize on the favorably changing age structure, they must play by the rules of solid economic behavior—not something that has previously characterized most LDCs. What sort of economic behavior? Entrepreneurial opportunity, open trading systems, deregulation, privatization, financial transparency, less corruption, sanctity of commercial contract law—all these proceeding in a humanitarian manner to offer protection to workers storm-tossed by a changing economic system. Easier said than done, but there is real evidence that it is beginning to happen in many LDCs. Further, the things we in the modern nations take for granted must be bolstered in the less developed nations: education, sanitation, public health, clean drinking water. If wealth can lead to health, the opposite is also true.

Aside from the formation of the demographic dividend, there are other factors at work that validate the idea of faster real per capita growth in the LDCs over the modern countries. Were it so, it would mean that over time, lots of time, the poor nations would catch up with the rich nations—economic convergence. This idea antedates the dividend theory.

Although most economists and developmental economists believe in convergence, and with some real surety, until recently it has not been easy to prove.* World Bank data, for example, shows that from 1971 to 1980, real per capita income growth for the LDCs was indeed higher than for the high income economies. But from 1981 to 1990, the modern nations were well higher than the LDCs. From 1991 to 2000, the growth rates were about the same.

World Bank forecasts for 2002 and 2003 show the LDC growth about twice as high as the modern nations. Moreover, World Bank

---

*The notion of "absolute" convergence in economic growth rates comes from the seminal theoretical work of Frank Ramsey (1928), Robert Solow (1956), and Trevor Swan (1956). But absolute convergence in economic growth has not been generally apparent in the cross-section data of countries. It requires (complicated) tests for "conditional" convergence to make the point, requiring (complicated) econometric regression analyses. For example, the empirical analysis by Robert Barro and Xavier Sala-I-Martin in their book *Economic Growth* (1995) suggests that economic growth rates tend to converge across countries, conditional on accounting for systematic differences in institutional factors and macroeconomic policy.

forecasts for 2004–2005 and 2006–2015 show LDC growth substantially higher than for the modern nations, roughly 3.4 percent to 2.2 percent, a significant difference.

(But who will get the new money? There is an argument, deeply enmeshed in the politics of LDCs, about "distribution." Is it just that the rich get richer and the poor stay poor? The same argument is to be heard in modern countries, including the United States. There are stacks of different data available to prove most any aspect of the distribution situation. In the United States, compensation packages of CEOs clearly soared relative to the wages of their employees. To a lesser extent there has been a widening gap between incomes of the well-to-do and the poor, albeit with a twist: the well-to-do got richer, but so did the poor, at a slower rate. It's hard to put a lot of new money in an economy and reserve it only for rich people; they do buy services from poor people. At best there is real redistribution happening in LDCs that had previously featured vast maldistribution.)

These World Bank numbers are nice to contemplate, but normally an economic forecast that goes as far out as 2015 would be considered dubious. In this case it looks quite reasonable. In 1991, the year India abandoned socialist state planning, the real national per capita growth rate was −1 percent. In the ensuing ten years, as market economics took hold, the growth rate was 4 percent per year. That's not bad, but not wildly exciting either. In the last few years, however, it appears as if India has begun to take off.

The big news is that India's fiscal year 2004 estimated a real annual GDP growth rate of 8.1 percent, compared to 4 percent the preceding year. India seems likely to continue boosting the global economy. In February 2004 the *Wall Street Journal*, in a major report on India's economy, quoted Mark Madden, manager of the Pioneer Emerging Funds, that "India looks like it is at the beginning of an 'upswing.'" (India's growth was boosted somewhat by favorable monsoons, the key to Indian agriculture.)

Beyond the demographic reasons cited in the Rand study, the World Bank projections, and the new Indian numbers, there are several other reasons to believe that the LDCs will grow more rapidly than the more developed nations.

First, the Indians and other LDCs are the beneficiaries of research work in the modern nations that took many years and much investment. Thus the Indian information technology boom was able to piggyback on costly investment originally done in America and other developed nations. So too with the exciting work India is now doing in biotechnology. Second, in the last few years India has benefited from a sharp increase in foreign investments, a point stressed in a very optimistic 2004 Salomon Smith Barney research report. (The SSB report also maintained that early elections in mid-2004 would give the present Indian government an opportunity for "tough reforms, corporate confidence, and stability." But, in a surprise, the government of Prime Minister Vajpayee lost to Sonia Ghandi's more government-oriented Congress party. After turning nervous on the news, the Indian stock market rebounded "after it became clear Congress would provide a stable government," according to the Associated Press. Then, in the following days, the market fell significantly and then rose again as the Communists in the likely Congress-led coalition announced that they too like foreign investment.)

Beyond this is the true "comparative advantage" available in the LDCs: cheap labor. In India's case, the labor force is not only inexpensive but often highly educated in fine schools. Inexpensive labor and good education, combined with foreign technology, research, and management, is a formula that yields healthy growth.

Economic convergence means that at some time in the future—admittedly the distant future—the earnings of the rich and poor countries will be about the same, or at least much closer to each other than is now the case. It should not be ignored by businessmen. It may well be the biggest economic story of the century. And, as we shall see later, it is also a hinge to another huge demographic story: immigration.

For all this to continue to happen, and to matter much, we must see continued fast growth in the two billionaire nations, China and India. It is not that the solid economic growth in, say, Thailand, with its population of 64 million people is not commendable, but the Thai population makes up only about 1 percent of the global total.

China and India, on the other hand, make up about 37 percent of the world's population. Both nations have enormous problems. Many American and foreign investors in recent decades have been burned by investments in what were called "emerging nations." But this may be the time for investors to make hay.

China is a Communist authoritarian nation with a generally robust capitalist economy. Will such a mixed bag prove politically stable? No one knows, but major political turmoil can play havoc with
an economy. China's official economic growth numbers are claimed to
average about 7 to 9 percent per year, numbers which are sensation-
ally high. But many cautious economists are mildly dubious, believing
the true rate is overstated by a percentage point or two. That would
still leave a sterling economic performance. In China, over the quarter-century from 1975 to 2000, per capita income soared from $273
per year to $3,976, as measured by "purchasing power parity."*

China's real per capita income in 2001 (in real exchangeable dollars this time as opposed to "purchasing power parity" as shown before) was about $900 per year. That's still a very low number, but
when multiplied by 1.3 billion people it yields more than a trillion
dollars per year, which could provide an important global economic
stimulus, particularly when coupled with the coming demographic
dividend.

India remains a poor country, much of it still populated by peas-
ants in dirt villages with primitive agriculture. It has a real per capita
income of about $500 per year. When real per capita income was
growing by close to 4 percent in the 1990s and early 2000s, the data
was regarded as more trustworthy than China's. At that time the annual growth added about $500 billion a year to the global GNP, com-
pounding on itself year after year. If the new growth rate continues,
that figure would roughly double. Of India's billion people, about
300 million are estimated to live in a middle-class urban situation—
roughly the total population of the United States. The Indian scientific and technical schools are something of a wonder of the world,
and Indians—in India and around the world—are among the leaders
of the global high-tech revolution. India may not yet be a global economic locomotive, but the wheels are moving.†

---

*"Purchasing power parity" represents the amount of goods and services that can
be purchased locally, as measured in dollars.

†Many oil experts ascribe part of the run-up in oil prices in early 2004 to increasing demand in China and India, not places normally regarded as huge consumer
markets. But it is now estimated that a thousand new cars come into use in Beijing
every day.

Other large LDCs with falling fertility rates also stand to cash in on the demographic dividend and help drive global economic growth. These include Bangladesh with 138 million people and a real 4.2 percent rate of per capita income growth in the 1990s.

One could write a book about investors who have lost their shirts in those emerging nations. Mistakes were made by most everyone concerned—investors, international organizations, the countries and the companies involved—often working under corrupt and inefficient regulations. I think the time has come for investors with a taste for risk to make their move in some of the LDCs. It would be a huge stroke of good fortune for the whole world in the decades to come.

IN DECEMBER 2003 the United Nations Population Division invited me to participate in another meeting of demographers and population experts from many countries. Once again the meeting was held in one of those elegant UN conference rooms equipped with translator booths, a place where the great issues of the day are discussed by the UN and sometimes resolved. This time, perhaps because of internal budget constraints, the meeting was held entirely in English. There were twenty-seven participants from many countries.

The meeting presented the assembled scholars with a draft report entitled "World Population in 2300." Three hundred years into the future is very far out indeed. Moreover, unlike the UNPD's previous 2150 projection, the new 2300 draft projected data by country, not just by continent.

The new document tried to reflect recent reality. In its press release it stated: "The new long-range population projections show a smaller future population size (9 billion persons) than previous United Nations long-range projections (10–12 billion). This is primarily due to the recent fertility declines occurring throughout the developing world and expectations that future fertility trends in the developing countries will follow the path experienced by the developed countries."

This approach is largely consistent with the demographic view I have presented here. First, there has been rapid fertility decline in the modern countries. Second, fertility rates in the LDCs have also fallen rapidly and will continue to fall. There is one exception: I believe that the world population totals will likely end up substantially lower than the 9 billion of the 2300 report and the 9 billion in 2050 of the Medium Variant 2002 projections.

The press release itself caused consternation among the experts. Its headline was "World's Population in 2300 to Be Around Nine Billion." Quite a number of the expert panelists rejected the tone of surety in the headline. They said no one knew what was going to happen three hundred years into the future, and in explaining the data the UNPD ought to be saying, "If such and such happens, this is how long-range population will look." The UN experts countered by noting that the tables in the new 2300 draft document were labeled "scenarios," not "projections," contrary to their earlier 2150 document.

Experts also complained that the document didn't really say anything new. Timothy Dyson of the Department of Population Studies at the London School of Economics noted that we already knew that population would be aging, that life expectancy would climb, and that dependency ratios would change.

As usual, the UN concentrated on its "Medium" scenario in the 2300 draft report. Its assumptions were quite interesting: the current UN baseline TFR of 1.85 children per woman would remain in place for a hundred years and then climb back to a global replacement rate—and, presumably, a stable population forever. I thought the most interesting observation at the meeting was offered by Paul Demeny of the Population Council in New York City. Demeny is of Hungarian origin. The TFR of Hungary is now 1.2 children per woman, and its population is projected to fall from 10 million in 2000 to 7.6 million in 2050, even if the Hungarian TFR should climb to 1.85 children per woman (a calculation that has no particular evidence today to back it up). Demeny asked, "What will we know in one hundred years that we don't know now that will boost fertility from 1.85 to 2.1?" Of course, no one had an answer.

I paid much of my attention to the "Low" scenario. With a few technical wiggles it is based on keeping the Total Fertility Rate at 1.85 children until 2300. Recall that a TFR of 1.85 is the *current* and *official* UN baseline total fertility rate announced with great fanfare in the 2002 *World Population Prospects*. (As explained earlier, that rate is substantially higher than current modern country rates, with no evidence yet supporting a reflation of fertility.) In any event, keeping that *current* and *official* UN baseline yields, in the "Low" scenario, a global population in 2300 of 2.3 billion people! That is quite different from the "Medium" scenario of 9.2 billion. At times like this it was the unique cast of Julian Simon's mind to ask if we might lose a Mozart or an Einstein in such a world. Or lose the woman who had the cure for cancer? Do you know? I don't. They were the kind of examples Simon would use to make people think.

Will population in 2300 move to 9 billion or to 2 billion? I do not know, and neither does anyone else. I lean toward the low side. All it requires is to follow the new UN baseline of 1.85 children per woman, should the TFR rise to that level in the modern nations and sink to that level in the poor countries.

Meanwhile, demographers from Mexico (Maria Elena Zuñiga Herrera of the Consejo Nacional de Población) and Brazil (Jose Alberto Magno de Carvalho) mentioned in passing that their countries had already fallen to the replacement rate, and they each expected further declines.

A final note for those interested in business conditions: keep your eyes open for changing demographics as the years go forward. The leverage in relatively small changes of fertility rates can mean that you will have fewer (or more) potential customers than you may be counting on. Granted, speculating about 2300 is pretty far out, but the shorter projections, particularly the ones for 2050 and 2025 presented here in words and charts, can be extremely valuable for farsighted businessmen. Never have birth and fertility rates fallen so far, so fast, so low, for so long, in so many places, so surprisingly.

CHAPTER TEN

The Environment

I AM SOMETIMES SKEPTICAL about what I see as exaggerations and crisis-mongering coming from the extremes of the environmental movement. But I tame my skepticism, or try to, when I recall a conversation I had a few years ago with Senator Joseph Lieberman.

Lieberman had been an activist attorney general in Connecticut before coming to serve in the U.S. Senate. He had been deeply involved in many environmental initiatives: clean air and water, wilderness preservation, and more. When he came to the Senate he continued on the green track. I asked him one day about his sometimes quite fervent environmental beliefs and statements. He is an observant Jew, and one senses that many of his political views derive from his belief in the divine. He paused for a brief moment, and said, "We are God's steward of nature."

We are indeed, or, if you are of a less theological cast of mind, we are nature's steward of nature. Clearly we have the ability to despoil much of nature's handiwork. We have demonstrated that unfortunate tendency in various ways and various places for thousands of years. So we have to be careful with our planet. Indeed, if one considers the political rhetoric of our time, we are all environmentalists now.

What does the New Demography and an examination of some ancillary facts tell us about our environmental future? A great deal. Since the reincarnation of active environmentalism in recent decades, two major thoughts have permeated environmental thinking.

The first is that people cause pollution. More people, doing whatever people do, means more pollution and more environmental degradation. When population was growing rapidly, this case was not hard to make. The numbers were staggering, with total world population peak figures, from the UN and other sources, coming in at 20 billion, 15 billion, and 11.5 billion by the UN in 1992. Now the properly computed number looks closer to 8 billion, a decrease of 3.5 billion people in just a decade.

The "global warming" debate has probably been the most publicized environmental issue of recent times. Of no small matter is the fact that the total global population of 11.5 billion was the base number used in the original global warming calculations that prompted such world concern.

But now we know something different. Human population is not exploding. According to the UN, global population will grow at a much lower rate than expected, then sink. We are likely in for an extended spell of depopulation. In the 1920s Oswald Spengler, in *The Decline of the West*, wrote that Europe's population would decline for two hundred years.

I take no adamant position, but I am somewhat skeptical about the great global warming scare, although most all atmospheric scientists agree there will be some warming. There is too much evidence to the contrary, pointing in too many directions and too often dismissed as "conservative rhetoric." Some examples: The largest part of the temperature increase in the twentieth century occurred in the first half of the century, not the second. Yet population growth and industrial activity was greater in the second half than in the first. Atmospheric weather satellites have shown only insignificant changes in recent decades. Data from weather balloons show a similar pattern. Moreover, if the problem is so severe, why don't environmentalists support nuclear power, which emits almost no greenhouse gases? In May 2004, writing in the UK's *Independent*, the British environmentalist James Lovelace made that suggestion and brought the house down upon his head.

The argument is bitter at times. In 2001 the Danish writer Bjorn Lomborg, a former environmental activist, caused a stir with his book *The Skeptical Environmentalist*. He wrote: "We are not running out of energy or natural resources. There will be more food per head of the world's population. Fewer and fewer people are starving." Here is more from Lomborg: "Global warming, though its size and future projections are rather unrealistically pessimistic, is almost certainly taking place . . . but the typical cure of early and radical fossil fuel cutbacks is way worse than the original affliction and, moreover, its total impact will not pose a devastating problem for our future."

In 2002 a group of scientists calling themselves the Danish Committee on Scientific Dishonesty reviewed Lomborg's heretical work and concluded: "Objectively speaking, the work under consideration is deemed to fall within the concept of scientific dishonesty." Yes, "dishonesty," a powerful word anywhere, particularly in scientific circles.

Then in late 2003 the Danish Ministry of Science, Technology, and Innovation not only cleared Lomborg of the charge of dishonesty but said the investigation of his work was sloppy and the charges "condescending and emotional." They further noted that the original committee didn't even allow Lomborg to present his case before the investigators.

Emotional rhetoric is not unusual in the environmental battle. In Albert Gore's 1992 book, *Earth in the Balance*, he writes things like this: Global warming "threatens an environmental holocaust. . . . Today the evidence of an ecological Kristallnacht is as clear as the sound of glass shattering in Berlin." Gore foresees the outbreak "of a kind of a global civil war" between the ecological "resistance fighters" and the "silent partners of destruction." Gore says opponents are "enablers" of such totalitarianism. Gore likes to point out that "the scientific argument about global warming is settled." Nonwarmist scientists are said to practice "junk science," like researchers who sell their souls to the tobacco industry.

But consider now *Beyond Malthus* (1999) by Lester Brown, Gary Gardner, and Brian Halweil, all of the Worldwatch Institute, of which Brown is president. Worldwatch is no marginal organization of green flakes. The book's introduction notes that Worldwatch is supported by some of the most important foundations in America, including Ford, Rockefeller Brothers, MacArthur, Hewlett Packard, Turner, Charles Stewart Mott, and, wouldn't you know, the UN Population

Fund. (Recall, that is not the professional demographic arm of the UN, the United Nations Population Division, whose work is cited throughout this book.)

Ignoring much demographic evidence, Brown argues that the world is suffering from "demographic fatigue," that the AIDS epidemic in sub-Saharan Africa is the leading indicator, and that it's all going to get worse unless we do what the book's authors say, immediately. What is this fatigue? What causes it? According to *Beyond Malthus*, the world's population is growing so fast in the less developed countries that there soon won't be enough grain, water, forests, fish, energy, jobs, housing, or meat. (As noted earlier, caloric intake in the LDCs, as measured by the UN's Food and Agriculture Organization, has gone up substantially.) Such demographic strains, say the authors of *Beyond Malthus*, are already raising death rates in sub-Saharan Africa, via AIDS. Birthrates may be falling now, but AIDS-like tragedies will increase birthrates, causing worse tragedy. Everyone everywhere ought to have condoms.

But one thing is clear about the case for global warming as seen by its advocates: human beings and their actions are causing the situation, and it is human beings who must reform their profligate ways. Accordingly, following the new UN data, we will have further growth (about two billion people) and then substantially fewer people than had been expected. And so we will first have more people-based pollution, though less than expected, and then much less pollution as populations shrink, causing less despoliation.

Part two of the environmental case is that affluence produces pollution. On the surface it makes sense. More pollution is created by those people driving SUVs and big cars, burning fuel in larger homes, carving up the wilderness for vacation homes, and so on. Beyond that is the matter of the destruction of the rain forest, the clear-cutting of forest land, strip mining, and other insults to nature.

But this cause-and-effect assumption is probably not the way the world works. We have data. During the years of the cold war, the free-market nations of Western Europe were vastly more industrialized, productive, and affluent than those in Communist Eastern Europe. Yet pollution of every sort—air, water, and ground—was vastly more extensive in the command economies of Eastern Europe.

Pollution levels in relatively affluent South Korea are much lower than in poor North Korea.

The same pattern is clear in the wealthy United States, a highly industrialized nation. Consider air pollution. The Environmental Protection Agency has been keeping records since 1976. Through 2001 the ambient air pollution levels for lead have dropped by 97 percent, carbon monoxide by 72 percent, sulfur dioxides by 67 percent, nitrogen dioxide by 42 percent, and ozone by 33 percent. Measurements levels for "particulates" (PM10) have been taken only since 1988; from that time to 2001 the level declined by 27 percent. All this happened while automobile travel grew by about 150 percent and the U.S. economy grew by 160 percent.*

The amount of forest land in America was stable from about 1920 to 1990, then increased from 1990 to 2002. We are not losing our natural habitat. The data for clean water points in a similar direction, though the data is not nearly as extensive. The percentage of American children exposed to unsafe water has declined from 20 to 8 percent just from 1993 to 1999. That is a 60 percent decline. The EPA monitors 650 chemicals for toxicity, a number that is up 40 percent in the last decade, while the level of toxic releases has declined by half.

A further argument about affluence is put forth by some activist environmentalists: as poor countries get wealthier, the population switches from a diet principally of grain to a protein diet with more meat, the production of which requires more environmental strain. Steven Hayward of the American Enterprise Institute maintains that there will be plenty of food to go around in the future. Although he thinks it is still an argument worth considering, he notes that the agricultural efficiencies of the Green Revolution have barely begun in some places. And, of course, it is worth restating that in a few decades the number of people to feed will be fewer.

Now, all these diminishments happened while American population was growing fairly rapidly. The 1975 population was 220 million. By 2000 it was 285 million, an increase of 30 percent.

*The material in this section comes principally from the "Index of Leading Economic Environmental Indicators, 2003," by Steven Hayward with Ryan Stowers (Pacific Research Institute for Public Policy and the American Enterprise Institute).

Why these environmental improvements? Because when a rich country decides to reduce pollution, it can do so, even as it grows richer. Part of the credit surely goes to the tumult raised by the environmental movement, notwithstanding its exaggerations. And a large part goes to the affluence that can be used for pollution-control measures.

Is America too crowded? Won't it be unbearably crowded when we add a projected 100 million people between 2000 and 2050?

Here is one happier scenario. American growth is coming principally from immigration. It will likely slow down over an extended period of time as fertility and then population decline in the "sending" nations, reducing the pool of prospective immigrants. Moreover, as noted in the preceding chapter, many of the poor are becoming more prosperous in their own countries, plausibly making emigration somewhat less attractive. The poor nations, remember, are getting richer faster than the rich nations, albeit from a much lower base. There will be a move toward global economic parity as the decades and centuries roll on. If people can make do in their own countries, most prefer not to uproot themselves and their families.

I find the environmental case to be mechanistic, almost robotic. Ever since the time of Malthus (and before), Malthusians have feared population growth: too many people chasing finite or depleting resources, chasing fewer or a finite number of jobs. But that's not the way it works. There is only one real resource: the intellect of man. In an atmosphere of liberty, it works overtime.

Four hundred years ago coal was a rock, relatively valueless. In the mid-nineteenth century, oil was still seen as gunk that fouled the streams of Pennsylvania. Few saw any value in uranium before the 1930s. Each became a "resource" when human ingenuity was applied. The human species is responsive. When cities fill up, suburbs form on the fringes. When suburbs fill up, we hear of "exurbs." Now demographers in the Western United States are talking about "leapfrog counties." If strip malls bother you, you can jump fifty miles and start a new place. It can happen most anywhere these days. A good phone system, access to roads, a computer hookup, a VCR, e-mail, cell phones, fax machines, and you're in business. As a matter of fact, the poorest places in America have been one of the greatest sources of population loss over recent years: the inner cities. And the wheel turns yet again: gentrification, "smart growth," and immigration begin to fill in formerly slum areas.

There is plenty of habitable land in America. We know that because it has been inhabited before. Small towns and big cities all over America are begging for new inhabitants to form new businesses with jobs. The infrastructure is mostly still in place. Moreover, if we choose, we often build up into the sky. People respond.

And people move. It is one of the powerful underlying strengths of the American economy that workers are willing to move when there are better jobs, or if they don't like their crowded areas. That has not been the European cultural pattern, which has much less mobility. Americans can be Americans anywhere in America. An Italian moving to Norway does not typically have such a feeling.

Let me return for a moment to the radio "phoners" after the publication of *The Birth Dearth*. The callers from places where population was falling—typically the American midcontinent—wanted more people. They said, "We're losing our young people." But many of the callers from places that were growing rapidly saw too many people and said, "Stop it." We won't be overcrowded in America because our freely elected legislators, from local to federal, zone the land. It is a line of work that too frequently gives birth to political scandal, but at the end of the day the results have not been bad. Parks and wilderness areas have been set aside all over the nation. (Rural population loss, with its environmental effects, is happening most everywhere. A German sociologist, Christine Hannemann, says, "People in East Germany are leaving in droves, and most of the ones leaving are young. Much of East Germany is turning into a series of ghost towns.") U.S. legislators have had little success in addressing the problem.

By any simple (and somewhat simplistic) measure, population density (the number of people per square mile) in the United States is way down in the rank order of nations. In 2001 America had 79 people per square mile. Yes, America has mountains, deserts, and Alaskan wilderness which are regarded as unhabitable. France, one of Europe's largest countries, has 283 people per square mile. Germany has 614 people per square mile. But, remember, those crowded nations are losing population and looking for ways to boost it.

Human beings respond to new conditions. Fertility and population grew rapidly as new medicines extended longevity in both the modern world and among the nations of the LDCs. Infants, in particular, lived longer. According to "demographic transition" theory, parents continued to have large families until they saw that their children really would live longer, providing heirs and rural child labor. Then fertility fell, dramatically.

So too will it be with the environmental problem. We will respond to conditions, whether that will involve zoning to prevent overcrowding, or adding people—probably immigrants—where people are needed and wanted. We are a responsive species. We'd better be.

CHAPTER ELEVEN

Geopolitics

PROBABLY MORE SO IN AMERICA than elsewhere, it is common to ask a new acquaintance, What do you do for a living? (It seems to be a question more often asked of and by men than of women, even in this time when large numbers of women are in the paid labor force.) From a geopolitical perspective, it is not an easy question to ask, or answer, about a nation, or a civilization.

The primary geopolitical job of America, and of most countries, is to defend itself. America's defense budget is about $450 billion per year, and expected to grow. Even so, during the war in Iraq, the American armed forces were said to be "stretched thin."

America's second job, I believe, is to vigorously promote social, economic, and individual liberty in America and around the world. Some of us believe it is not an either-or proposition. Promoting liberty helps defend America. And, as I see it, there is no better inheritance to pass along to posterity. You only live once; do something with your life.

The idea that America is, and should be, enthusiastically involved in the global promotion of liberty is an arguable proposition. But such is my view. I believe that in its modern incarnation, at least in America, the notion stems in serious measure from the neo-conservative movement. As an early and vocal neo-con, I might be able to write a book about it. I will spare you. But there are demographic implications to the current situation of liberty in the world that deserve to be examined.

The course of global liberty-promotion has traversed a bumpy track in America. Yes, slavery was legal in America; yes, unpardonable sins were visited on American Indians. But social and economic liberty has been moving in a salutary direction for several centuries. The evidence of recent decades strongly suggests that liberty-promotion has become a worldwide cause, in fact the preeminent one today. That cause, as we shall see, is one aspect of the current fight against the number one geopolitical problem of our time, the threat of mass terror.

Given such a stipulation—that defense and the extension of liberty are America's principal geopolitical goals—what are the effects of the New Demography? It is a question that takes us through some tangled thickets.

Of course demographics have always played a powerful role in the games nations play. In the past, a nation with more people was perceived to have a major military advantage over a potential adversary with fewer people.

That idea has a long history dating back to ancient times. From *Newsweek* of November 2003: "He is politely called the god of 'fertility,' but the Egyptian deity Min had a lot more on his mind than agriculture. Invariably depicted with a large erect penis, he was the God Pharaoh would pray to when he needed Egyptian women to conceive more soldiers for his army, and his favorite offering was lettuce, considered a powerful aphrodisiac by the ancient Egyptians."

The first half of the twentieth century was a time when this demographic linkage to warfare was clearly believed. In the late nineteenth and early twentieth centuries, demographic calculations showed that the Germans had substantially higher fertility rates than the French. In a world of trench warfare, needing huge armies to serve as "cannon fodder," such data could produce fear of occupation, which could prompt an arms race, which could yield war. Adolf Hitler's demonic call for demographic *lebensraum* was in just such a tradition. (Today, ironically, the numbers are quite different. The German TFR is 1.35 children per woman; the French TFR at 1.89 is more than half a child higher.)

The demographic data we deal with here are a long way from being fully comprehensive, but as we scan the future geopolitical canvas, one question stands out: Will the old geopolitical rules from a world in which the number of people had been growing for centuries still apply to one where the number of people is already shrinking rapidly in many places and is scheduled to shrink most everywhere later in this century?

Consider war, the plague of the human species. Wars can have many causes, but from earliest times nations have sought to conquer land in order to accommodate more people and gain control of more resources. What happened in the first half of the twentieth century might serve as a model of those factors in play.

In the future, broadly speaking, there will be more population pressure in the LDCs as the world grows from about 6 billion to about 8 billion by 2050. But that is a much slower growth rate than we have seen in the last fifty years. So while there may be more people with war on their minds, they will be appearing at a slower rate, perhaps less inclined to believe they need an invasion or two to make things right. After that, population sinks, in theory further reducing the perceived need for war.

And then there is the European-Soviet case. The peaceful dismemberment of the Soviet Union must surely be counted as one of the great events of our time. There are still instabilities, to be sure, but the two great nuclear powers are not thinking about MAD (Mutual Assured Destruction) anymore. And both Russia and the European nations are in steep demographic decline, with fewer potential soldiers and less ability to fight conventional wars.

CAN THE NEW DEMOGRAPHY tell us much about the future of our favorite civilization, that is, Western civilization?* In fact, I believe it can.

We begin with some items about which there is little argument. In the next half century or so, Western civilization will become an ever-smaller fraction of total world population. In 1950, the point at which the current UN statistical series begins, the percent of the

---

*Which, in this analysis, coincides with the UN's "More Developed Regions" category rather than excluding Japan as Samuel Huntington does in *The Clash of Civilizations*.

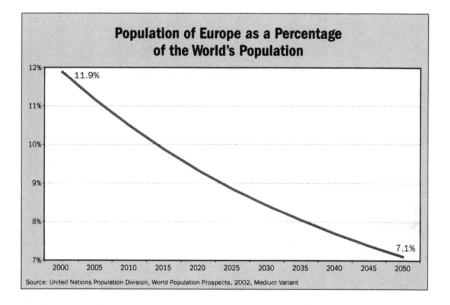

Population of Europe as a Percentage of the World's Population

11.9%

7.1%

Source: United Nations Population Division, World Population Prospects, 2002, Medium Variant

world that was in the Western civilization club was at 32 percent. But by the year 2000, after an LDC population explosion, the proportion was 20 percent. In 2050, as estimated by the UN Medium Variant, the proportion of "The West" to "The Rest" is projected to be 14 percent. These are the numbers that should be drilled into our head if we want to consider the Western demographic impact on the geopolitical future: 32, 20, 14 percent, and sinking. In a hundred years, from 1950 to 2050, the West will fall from about one-third to about one-seventh of world population.

The European numbers, as opposed to those for all the West, are even more dramatic. (See the chart above.) Europe had a global population share of 22 percent in 1950, 12 percent in 2000, and is projected to be at 7 percent in 2050. In the hundred years from 1950 to 2050, Europe will have fallen from somewhat more than one-fifth of the world's people to about one-twelfth. The demographer Paul Demeny estimates that for every 1,000 Europeans in the year 2000, there will only be 232 in the year 2100.

America, growing, will just about hold its own in the years when LDC fertility is shrinking, but from a high base. In 1950 the United States made up 6.3 percent of the global population. In 2000 it had fallen to 4.7 percent. In 2050 the UN "Medium" projection is for 4.6 percent and actually moving up slightly.

Demographically, the West is not doing well overall. Except for America, it is doing very poorly. The Western plunge is led by Europe and Japan with those astonishing 1.3 and 1.4 TFRs. But it is important to note that while the West has not been the largest demographic grouping in a very long time, the modern West has been the most powerful, most affluent, most technologically proficient civilization in history. Demography matters, a great deal, but obviously many other factors come into play. And the Westerners have managed to accomplish their sterling deeds while periodically taking time off to slaughter one another in the most devastating wars of history.

Still, we have now seen sixty years of general peace among the Western European nations. That is a remarkable human achievement. Today it is just about inconceivable that members of the European Union or NATO would send young men into battle to kill each other. There has been progress, real progress, that would have been almost unimaginable in the middle of the twentieth century.

High-profile arguments are not uncommon among the nations of the West. The war in Iraq showed how bitter and important those arguments can be. But in looking at the modern world, one should not forget that the Western nations share critical and common values even in times of dispute. All are democracies; their citizens vote for their leaders. They have a free press. Workers have a right to organize independent of the government. An independent judiciary shares power with the government. The West is a real civilization with broad and deeply held common values. (Of course, the United States would not be allowed to join the European Union because some American states allow the death penalty. On the other hand, public opinion polls show majorities in some European nations support the death penalty.)

While the United States is generally regarded today as the sole superpower, there are fads and fashions in geopolitics as well as changing realities. And they can be products of demographics. For a flavor of these arguments, and how they change, let us take a detour to consider the somewhat strange intellectual hegira of Yale's Paul Kennedy.

His best-selling book *The Rise and Fall of the Great Powers* appeared in 1988. In it he predicted that America as a great power

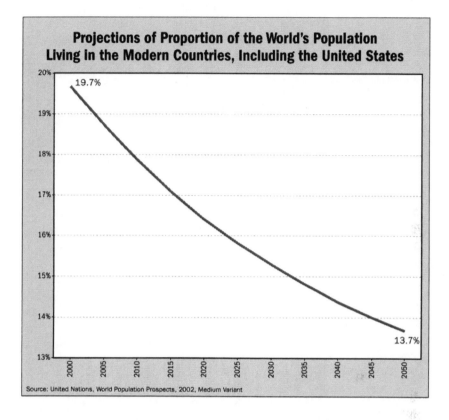

Projections of Proportion of the World's Population Living in the Modern Countries, Including the United States

19.7%

13.7%

Source: United Nations, World Population Prospects, 2002, Medium Variant

would fall victim of what he called "imperial overstretch." Americans, he said, should begin planning a foreign policy that would enable it to manage its decline gracefully. Kennedy, and others, mocked American "triumphalism," a word much in use after the fall of the Soviet Union. (I was, and am, a triumphalist, albeit always nervous about it. You never know what comes next.)

Indeed, if such a graceful decline had to be accomplished, that was a pretty good time to write finis to the great American experiment and the notion of a global Pax Americana. America did not have a good run from the early 1970s to the early 1980s. In 1975, *Commentary* magazine, a haven for hawkish neo-conservatives, printed a long symposium entitled "America Now: A Failure of Nerve?"

The tragedy in Vietnam so split the nation that even hawks wondered if the United States had lost its somewhat messianic bent. It was said that Vietnam and Watergate had sapped the American spirit (an obscene formulation, coupling a war that killed millions with a president who lied). The American inflation rate had soared to a thirty-three-year high of 13.5 percent in 1981. Interest rates didn't peak until they reached 19 percent in January that year. Economic growth had pretty well stalled. Crime was rising. Out-of-wedlock birth was climbing. In the classic barometric polling question of "right-track, wrong-track," Americans in the early 1970s responded by rates of about 7 to 1 that the nation was on the "wrong track." By 1983 the "wrong track" respondents were still dominant by rates of about 2 to 1.* President Jimmy Carter never actually used the word "malaise" in that famous speech, but that's what it was about.

America withdrew from South Vietnam without a victory and with a treaty that was betrayed by the North Vietnamese before the ink was dry. To some, the Soviets, as well as other totalitarians, seemed to be the wave of the future. Hawks were in anguish. Communists, they said, were taking over in Nicaragua, Angola, Cambodia, and Afghanistan. Might American values no longer be the face of the future? According to many conservatives, liberals were questioning the whole American global enterprise. There was a fear that isolationism would return to America.

And all the while there was Japan. That was Paul Kennedy's model. It seemed the Japanese could do no wrong. Over the decade of the 1970s and through 1989 the Japanese annual growth rate, discounted for inflation, was 4.6 percent—very strong for a modern nation over an extended period of time. At that rate the Japanese Gross Domestic Product would double in just fifteen years. It wouldn't be long before Japan would overtake America in per capita income.

Truly better Japanese automobiles were cutting into sales of American-made vehicles. Japanese television sets and electronic gadgetry were at the cutting edge. Its work force was disciplined. Americans were treated to video clips of Japanese workers exercising in the morning while singing the company anthems of Japan's powerhouse

---

*Data from the Roper Center. In 1983 the leading causes of discontent were "a letdown in moral values," "permissiveness in the courts," and, significant for the argument here, "too much commitment to other nations in the world." In the world of survey research, concerns about defense seem to rise to high levels only when the threat is great and clear.

industrial corporations. And it was, we were told, all part of a grand plan, much of it set in motion by a government agency, the Ministry of International Trade and Industry.

Japan would be Number One! And near Japan were the "Four Tigers"—Taiwan, Hong Kong, South Korea, and Singapore. They too were growing rapidly and capturing large pieces of the American market.

That was the future Paul Kennedy saw. He maintained that America just couldn't compete with Nippon and the Tigers. We weren't even doing well compared to the Europeans. We wouldn't be Number One. We didn't even have a plan. Our workers were lazy. And, after all, civilizations rise and civilizations fall. (As Casey Stengel said, "That's a true fact.")

Kennedy examined the British, French, Dutch, Portuguese, and Roman empires. They all rose, they all fell. Now it was America's turn. The Europeans were so sad about America's plight. Jacques Attali, then the head of the European Bank of Reconstruction and Development, balefully wrote that "America had become Japan's 'granary,' like Poland was for Flanders in the seventeenth century." Kennedy trumpeted that America's share of the global GDP was "only" about 22 percent and had been steadily declining from 30 percent since the end of World War II.

(But much of this was to be expected; Japan and the European nations had been devastated by World War II and had grown rapidly from their destroyed base. Although about 400,000 Americans were killed in World War II, and many more injured, the war was basically fought in Europe and in Pacific lands, not on American soil. Many parts of Europe and Japan were effectively obliterated. They had a lot of catching up to do from a very low base, often starting from Ground Zero. In any event, for one nation out of about 200 to account for more than one-fifth of global economic activity was in any event quite remarkable.)

By my lights, Kennedy's thinking was well off the mark. But James Fallows, Clyde Prestowitz, and many other "declinists" wrote about it at length, engendering much comment and even some action in the policy community. A book and movie by Michael Crichton showed murderous Japanese thugs at work undermining American industry.

Why was such thinking wrongheaded even then?

It is wrongheaded to suggest that being Number One is the same as being the wealthiest. For a while, when oil prices were high, Kuwait had the highest per capita income in the world. They were not Number One. They were not a superpower, sole or otherwise.

Military strength isn't everything, but no nation whose defense is provided by another nation can even dream of being Number One. For many years during the cold war, the United States was spending about four times more than Japan on defense, proportional to population, or about eight times as much in total. America's nuclear shield and global fleet protected Japan from very dangerous neighbors, the Soviet Union and China.

The four famous tigers were then under a de facto American security umbrella. Hong Kong was officially "defended" by its British colonial status, but Britain was half a world away and had difficulty dispelling several hundred Argentines from the Falkland Islands, let alone defending Hong Kong from the mainland Chinese Communists should they choose to take it over. (The Chinese later legally reclaimed Hong Kong peacefully, as if the Brits could have stopped them even if they chose to.) Through NATO, America provided much of the defense shield for Western Europe.

A Number One influential nation must have a vast cultural reach. But around the world there were relatively few Japanese movies, books, or magazines that achieved popular global eminence. Japanese was not taught as a mandatory second language elsewhere in the world. By contrast, in many places around the world English was routinely taught to schoolchildren as a language requirement. American music, global journalism, television, movies, science, and education were dominant most everywhere. American cultural potency—what Harvard's Joseph Nye calls "soft power"—played a mighty role in shaping the way the world lives.

And, most important from a demographic perspective, it would be difficult to maintain that a nation on a path to severe population decline might be seriously considered as Number One. Even as Kennedy and the American declinists were preaching American failure and Japanese supremacy, the Japanese fertility rate had already fallen well below replacement, to 1.81 children per woman in 1975–

1980. In the 1980–1985 time frame the rate fell to 1.76. By 1985–90 the rate was 1.66, then 1.49. The 2002 rate was 1.32. In mid-June 2004 the Japanese government announced the 2003 rate at 1.29.

The Japanese demographic story is an interesting one. Following the catastrophic wartime experience of the Japanese, a very brief baby boom ensued. From 1950 to 1955 the Japanese TFR was 2.75. But by the next five-year time frame (1955–1960) the TFR was just below replacement (2.08), and there it remained for twenty years.

The echo effect from Japan's short-lived post–World War II baby boom produced some population growth even as fertility rates tumbled. Japan's population in 1975 was 112 million. By the year 2005 (roughly now) the Japanese population had grown to 128 million, an increase of 15 percent over thirty years. (The U.S. population grew by 35 percent during the same period.)

But momentum-induced Japanese population growth has now just about stopped, and Japan is slated for a decline from 128 million to 105 million by 2050 (using the Constant-Fertility Variant projection), a decrease of 17 percent, with more shrinkage to come. Moreover, Japan is a relatively small island, no larger than the size of California. Such a nation was not about to lead the world because it made the best cars, which it did and probably still does.

With all that, many American economic analysts believed in the idea of Japanese economic supremacy. Indeed, Japan had a remarkable half-century of growth. More important, many Japanese thinkers believed it. It is not a country without a history of smug cultural supremacy. James Fallows, writing in the June 22, 1987, issue of *U.S. News and World Report*, quoted the Liberal party chairman Noboru Takeshita as joking at a political rally that "the ever-rising yen had made American sailors stationed in Japan too poor to afford Japanese bar girls . . . the lonely sailors only alternative was to stay on base and give each other AIDS."

But Japan did not have a good decade in the 1990s, nor did it do well in the first few years of the new century. There were recessions; there was a very sluggish economy. Economic analysts studied the "Japanese Disease" and wondered about a true economic crash. In the late 1990s Asia was swept into massive economic turmoil due principally to "overbuilding," or so it was said. The Thai economy got into trouble; Malaysia suffered; the Indonesian economy and polity came close to collapse; the "Asian Contagion" swept across the area. These are doughty nations, and for the most part they have bounced back. But they don't much remind one of the steady and glorious ascendant path that Paul Kennedy had sketched out for them. One might guess that today Kennedy is advising the Japanese to manage their decline gracefully.

Foreign journalists had a better take on what was happening. I was a member of President Lyndon Johnson's staff during the latter part of the 1960s. I traveled to many foreign countries with Johnson. Every report in the host nation press began the same way: "President Lyndon Johnson, the most powerful man in the world, today arrived in . . ." Later presidents have been treated the same way, despite whatever disputes were in progress. It is not a sentence written about the Japanese prime minister when he travels abroad.

In any event, Paul Kennedy changed his mind—sort of. It was not what happened on 9/11 that did it. It was what happened *after* 9/11 that turned Kennedy's head. Writing at length in the *Financial Times*, he limned a different picture of America.

The U.S. aircraft carrier *Enterprise* was in the Indian Ocean at the time. Immediately it began steaming toward the action in Afghanistan. Kennedy tells us about the carrier *Enterprise*. I have spent a few days on an American carrier and have had a taste of its naval grandeur; but it was the *USS Forrestal*, an older, smaller ship. The *Enterprise* was a newer vessel, and there are still others coming on line. Kennedy reported breathlessly that the *Enterprise* was as high as a 20-story building and almost as long as four football fields. A crew of 5,600 men and women see to it that the ship's 70 planes can fly missions day or night, in weather calm or stormy.

Moreover, Kennedy informed us, an American carrier travels in a "carrier battle group" which includes Aegis-class cruisers to shoot down incoming missiles; a screen of destroyers and frigates to defend against submarines; killer-submarines; supply ships; and Marine troops with their helicopters ready for combat. Kennedy estimated that the cost of a complete carrier battle group amounted to about one-quarter of the defense budget of an entire medium-size country. America had twelve such carrier groups. And there was no competition, Kennedy noted: "The few UK, French, and Indian carriers are minuscule by comparison, the Russian ones rusting away." In short, America was the only nation in the world that could project its power and destroy targets anywhere in the world.

Kennedy, the same man who wrote about America's "imperial overstretch," noted that America was militarily powerful "on the cheap." In the 1960s military costs had amounted to about 9 percent of America's GDP. By 1985, as a post-Vietnam America had begun to "reorder its priorities," the proportion was 6 percent. Today, even after 9/11 and with the ensuing military buildup, the share of America's GDP going to the military is about 4 percent.

This time around, Kennedy did not neglect America's soft power. He stressed Nobel laureates, its superior universities, the biggest banks, the biggest companies, the spread of the English language, the movies, television, advertising, international student flows, and so on and on.

Kennedy is a numbers cruncher. He notes that back when America produced a (mere) 22 percent of the world's GDP, and that share was declining, it was an indicator of America's continuing fall. He states in his 2002 article that "Had this decline continued for another decade or two, America would have come troublingly close to imperial overstretch." (Kennedy did not bother to tell his readers that it was he who was leading the overstretch charge.)

In any event, as Kennedy notes, things have changed. The Soviet Union collapsed. Japan's amazing economic growth stalled. American businessmen made their companies leaner and meaner, producing sharp gains in productivity. Kennedy notes that America no longer produces 22 percent of world GDP but is back to about 30 percent. In short, the United States is not only the single surviving superpower but the most powerful and influential nation in world history. And Kennedy says it will likely remain so for the foreseeable future. (Given Kennedy's track record, that is a prediction I would worry about.)

Has Kennedy simply reversed field? Not quite. As he states: "America's present standing very much rests upon a decade of impressive economic growth. But were that growth to dwindle, and budgetary and fiscal problems to multiply over the next quarter of a century, the threat of overstretch would return." Profound: if over-stretch returns there will be overstretch.

If the generally ascendant path of global economic growth contin-ues for another twenty-five years (or fifty years, for that matter), Amer-ica will remain the most powerful economic force in the world, albeit not by proportionately as much as now. The large LDC nations— China and India most importantly—are growing their economies at a faster rate, and they will be adding more producers than the United States. But it will be a very long time, with many imponderables sure to rise up, before the large LDCs "catch up" to America. (Although one Chinese businessman was quoted in 2004 as saying that the Chi-nese yuan would be the world's "reserve currency" by 2050.)

Kennedy's wool-gathering about overstretch and America's geopolitical role in the world is off the mark in at least two major ways, both linked to demographics.

To have a large and powerful military force requires a great deal of money. The American military budget for fiscal year 2005 is esti-mated to be near $450 billion per year. Where does the money come from? Military spending is generally a fixed expense. These days the American elected government has determined we need that $450 bil-lion per year to face our current defense needs. Given our perception of a dangerous global situation, we would need about that much money whether our population were 200 million or 300 million. With a larger population, the cost per person goes down; there is an economy of scale at work. That is one reason the United States has been able to meet its perceived military needs. With the 400 million people expected by 2050, we should continue to be able to meet our perceived needs. Some recent estimates show that the United States is spending about as much money on its military as all other nations combined!

By contrast, population figures provide one reason why Euro-peans will likely have to cut their defense spending in the decades to come. In the case of a nation with a declining population, the cost per person for fixed expenses goes up as the population goes down. More young people, many of them immigrants, means that the United States can easily get by with no need to seriously consider a military draft, which some European nations still maintain.

During the cold war, Republicans, hawks, and "Reagan Democrats" believed that liberal Democrats did not fully appreciate the
global expansionary potential of the Soviet Union, and that they were
"soft on defense." Democrats still regard "soft on defense" as their
major political weak spot. Republicans, particularly after 9/11, continue to play that string on the national political fiddle. But that is
politics. America has plenty of money for defense, and there is little
doubt that attention to it will continue. As a general matter, when the
next Democratic president is elected he or she will make sure America has enough for its defense, and America will continue to feel a
deep responsibility to bolster and extend liberty.

Americans should remember that the stakes are immense. America seeks to lead the world to those "broad sunlit uplands" that Winston Churchill talked of during World War II, uplands characterized
by liberty. It will not be an easy task. It will be especially difficult if
the Europeans, who are in their own way fine exemplars of liberty,
are not wholeheartedly on our side. To try to keep them on our side,
America should bend over backward whenever possible to soothe the
Europeans. After all, the Europeans are a demographically diminishing band of nations. We should treat them well and stop the French-
frying, tempting as it may be.

HOW IS DEMOGRAPHY related to the second part of America's mission, the extension of democracy and individual liberty?

We should note first that democratic values, both civil and economic, have been in the ascendancy around the world. The index
compiled by Freedom House shows that in 1973 there were *forty-
three* "free states" and sixty-nine "not free." Thirty years later there
were *eighty-nine* "free" states and forty-eight "not free," a huge re-
versal. (Freedom House also categorizes states as "partly free.")
Among the criteria Freedom House requires for a country to make
the "free" list are free and fair elections, with opposition political
parties allowed to operate freely; freedom of expression, including
an uncensored media; freedom of religious practice; an independent
judiciary; freedom to travel within the nation; and freedom for
unions to operate and organize. Joshua Muravchik of the American
Enterprise Institute adds that these liberties must be available to all.

During the rule of apartheid, South Africa had many of the these freedoms—for whites only.

The *Wall Street Journal* and the Heritage Foundation compile a similar index of "economic freedom" (in other words, free-market economics). Although the data have been compiled over a much shorter time frame, a similar trend is apparent. In 1995, 6 countries ranked as "free" and 35 ranked as "mostly free," a total of 41 of the 101 nations surveyed. In 2003 there were 15 countries ranked "free" and 56 ranked "mostly free," a total of 71 of the 156 nations surveyed. That's still a minority, but the increase over just eight years is solid. Among the criteria weighed in the survey are level of taxation, trade and tariff policy, government expenditures as a percent of Gross Domestic Product, and freedom to set prices privately without government influence and smuggling.

By any historical standard, social and economic liberty is on the march as never before. The goal is liberty, not, as sometimes charged, "a bunch of little Americas around the world." This freedom is clearly related to income. Among low-income countries, 16 percent are fully free, including Mali, Ghana, Benin, Senegal, Angola, Lesotho, the Philippines, and the world's largest democracy, India.

This free and democratic surge has been led by America through both governmental and nongovernmental means. Americans spent huge amounts of government money during the cold war to contain the threat of a nuclear-armed Soviet Union. It was money earmarked for military purposes. But its real rationale was to defend a way of life for ourselves and our allies, and to protect against the possibility of Soviet global expansion.* Beyond that America sought to extend the precepts of such a way of life to nations around the world.

The Harvard and Cambridge scholar Amartya Sen was asked what was the most important event of the twentieth century. As he

---

*America regarded Eastern European nations as invaded by the Soviets. In 1959 the United States declared "Captive Nations Week" to emphasize the fact that the Eastern Europeans were not a group of acquiescent socialists. While the satellite nations had Soviet troops on their soil, they were ruled by Communist "puppet" regimes, albeit not directly from Moscow. "Captive Nations Week" is still declared each year by the president, as it was in 2003, with the Eastern Europeans off a list that is now expanded to note the lack of human rights in countries such as Burma, Iran, North Korea, Zimbabwe, and Belarus.

recounts it, he ran through his mind the fall of the empires, the great wars, the rise and fall of communism, and many other great events. And he concludes, "I did not, ultimately, have any difficulty in choosing one as the preeminent development of the period: the rise of democracy."* Sen also notes that the rise of democracy as we know it today is a new phenomenon. Of course it had its roots in ancient Greece, the Magna Carta, the American and French revolutions. But only now, Sen writes, has "the idea of democracy become a universal value."

I believe this is so, and that it is a blessing given the demographic data showing that the Western democracies will be only a very small portion of the world's population. For our own benefit, we should encourage more of the Less Developed Countries to become democratic, and for those who already make the cut list, to become more democratic. Most of them, after all, are newcomers to the process. They need all the help they can get. Further, the new democracies are mostly poor nations. Again, for our own benefit, we should do all that we can to make the LDCs more prosperous. It is fairly clear that democracy boosts prosperity and prosperity boosts democracy.

There is yet another aspect of self-interest. Liberty-promoters make an important nondemographic point which we should consider. Democratic nations do not go to war with one another.† And when wars break out, America, as the sole superpower, too often gets involved, with blood or treasure, or both.

I don't think I have ever seen a poll that did not show "foreign aid" very far down the list of popular federal spending programs. Karlyn Bowman, the survey expert at the American Enterprise Institute says, "In polls conducted over the past several decades at least, 'foreign aid' tends to be very unpopular. It is seen as helping foreigners, not Americans, and it is likely that many people think the money is not well spent." But sometimes leadership must trump political popu-

---

*Journal of Democracy, July 1999.
†There may be an exception to prove the rule. In 1948 Lebanon, a mostly democratic nation, participated in the Arab League's war against democratic Israel. But Lebanon was the smallest and weakest of the Arab states. It voted against the war in League meetings but was more or less compelled to go along. A few weeks after the fighting began, Lebanon surrendered.

larity. If America is to lead a global crusade for liberty, we had better be prepared to spend more money to help the people we hope will join the effort. If some of the money is corruptly diverted, so be it. As it is, we give a smaller proportion of our GDP to poor nations than most European countries. (That is a little more complicated than it appears. Millions of immigrants in America send huge amounts of money to their families back home. Unlike much government-to-government or institutional foreign aid, this money is rarely tainted with official corruption.) Estimates on remittances vary, but the amount is believed to be $30 billion to Latin America alone, according to an Inter-American Development Bank report issued in mid-2004.

ALL THIS should sound familiar to American and Western readers. Western civilization, led by the United States, has given birth to a global culture. It has many flaws, but it is as good as measurable humanity gets. (The UNPD does not measure human happiness, only the absence of human misery, which is no small matter.)

The progress we have seen toward liberty has probably come about more from private American sources than from public ones. The global distribution of American movies and television has shown the American way of life to all, including its tawdry aspects. American music, rock 'n' roll and successor genres, has captivated audiences around the world. Sending a man to the moon demonstrated American technological power, as did stunning American developments in high-tech industries. American books have a global market, as do many American magazines and several daily American newspapers. And individual immigrants continue to tell their families what life is like in America.

All this, by now, is no longer driven by official America. It probably never was. There are plenty of Americans—right, left, and center—who think we have veered off course, culturally or geopolitically, and that we should stop the freedom crusade. But such, I believe, is the role history has assigned us in this remarkable moment, whether we like it or not.

Are there threats to this largely salutary human development? Are there demographic answers to such threats?

There is, first, the front-page story of our moment: terrorism. At its root it is an attack on Westernism and modernism—and America is the Great Satan of Westernism. Osama bin Laden and Al-Qaeda regard individual liberties as their sworn enemies. Long term, nothing could play better into the hands of the Islamist radicals than to see the Western world shrink of its own accord. (Some of the radicals have boasted of the high Muslim rates of demographic growth, which, as we have seen earlier, is a complicated issue but with some real truth to it.)

Terror is an old technique and will never be entirely eradicated. But over the long term terrorism may be diminished in a major way only when the peoples of the terrorist states turn vigorously on the terrorists. That is more likely to happen as and if democratic values spread among the peoples residing in states that sponsor terrorism, or in states that are afraid to fight it. People who are able to run their own affairs do not like it when their societies are terror-bombed. All the more reason to go about our democracy-building pursuits.

On the demographic side, we can only shudder to think what would happen to the Western experiment in liberty if the entire Western population continued to shrink. At least America will grow. Roughly speaking, in the next half-century the modern democratic nations, not counting the United States, will lose well over 100 million people, depending on whose estimates are used. Meanwhile, America is projected to grow by at least that same figure.

It's hard for me to imagine that the advance of individual and economic liberties in the world would continue without an exemplar nation that is prospering and growing. In the modern world America is that nation. It is the place where the world's people will look to see if the great democratic experiment continues to flourish. Were America on the European/Japanese track of population decline, the case for democracy would be much harder to make. Imagine, for example, that instead of growing from 300 million to more than 400 million people, the United States were to reproduce in the European mode and lose 50 million people in the next 50 years, ending up at about 250 million people. It would be a world without a clear exemplar of a growing and successful democratic model.

Yet this mix of a large and powerful population and a belief system of individual freedom has also made America target number one in the terrorist cross hairs.

Demographics have played a central role in our current situation. After many decades of high immigration, the United States in 1924 passed highly restrictive immigration laws designed to keep out potential Americans who were not of a Northwestern European heritage. Among the proponents of the restrictions was the Ku Klux Klan. In 1965 new, more liberal legislation was passed. But what if American immigration had been pretty well cut off in 1824. Or suppose for some other reason that America had not grown to be a populous nation of 300 million people, with more than another 100 million expected in the next 50 years. Suppose instead that the population of the United States today was somewhere in the range of Japan (127 million) or Russia (146 million). Suppose, in short, that America today was somewhat less than half as populous as it is.

Would such an America be the world's "sole superpower"? I doubt it. It would be a nation with somewhat less than half the Gross Domestic Product it now has, and less able to use its financial power in instances when such power can be used in America's interest. It might still have the world's most potent military but not by the margins it now enjoys. Tax revenues to support the military would be halved, or costs to taxpayers doubled. Military expenditures would probably be cut sharply.

Such a situation would likely encourage the growth of competitor states, which is precisely what all those policy memoranda from the National Security Council and the Department of Defense seek to discourage. In somewhat more technical language, those official documents state that America intends to be Number One, with no qualifications. With half its current population, and shrinking in the European fashion, that would be a dubious proposition.

Returning to the American reality, we nonetheless must look forward to competitors in the twenty-first century. A glance at the demographic map shows who the big players in the modern world are.

Europe. Under normal circumstances, a united Europe in some form might be one such potential competitor. It is rich. Aggregated, its many nations are more populous than America. But Europe will be losing population sharply and will accordingly be losing military and commercial power. It is a continent still divided politically. It took America to bail Europe out of a relatively small mess in the former Yugoslavian states. The situation may change, but for the foreseeable future "assertive" would not likely be an adjective to associate with the union of European states.

Still, Europe is a big, rich place. It will decline from 728 million people in the year 2000 to 597 million in 2050. But 600 million people with democratic values, slowly opening a unified economy, cannot be dismissed. In 2050 Europe will still be much more populous than the United States, although if Eastern Europe is excluded it will soon be a close match. Despite tensions between the two, America and Europe usually take the same side on major issues. As we shall see, both are members of what some call "the Liberty party," and that's the big one.

Russia. Russia remains a puzzle, feared by many of its neighbors. But it too is losing population, and it is a diseased nation. It would seem that the Russian Federation has decades of domestic rebuilding as its first priority.

India. India will become the largest nation in the world in a few decades. It deserves a permanent seat on the UN Security Council. Its per capita income is growing sharply, but from a very low base. It is a nation with nuclear weapons and a strong reputation in military circles. It faces regional conflict (with Pakistan) but has not entered global politics in a major way.

India is the world's largest democracy and has been for more than half a century. As long as it remains democratically governed it will most likely be a geopolitical ally of the United States on major issues, not likely a competitor. It gives the lie to the idea that some nations or some peoples aren't "ready" for democracy.

If India presents any challenge to America, it is because its work in information technology is so expert that it is taking American jobs. A *Business Week* article suggests that India "will be the first developing nation that used its brainpower, not natural resources or the raw muscle of factory labor, as a catalyst." Demographically, the report notes, India's economic growth "is inspiring more of the best and brightest to stay home rather than migrate." A twenty-four-year-old Indian graduate in information technology put it this way: "We work in world-class companies, we're growing, and it's exciting . . . the opportunities exist here in India."

Of course, India has great problems too—poor roads, slums piled with garbage heaps, migrants sleeping on bare pavement, illiteracy, and bureaucracy. There is also an HIV/AIDS threat to be concerned about. Across the river from Calcutta is Howrah, the grimmest slum I have ever seen.

Meanwhile the fall in Indian fertility rates continues. Of the five main states in the southern part of the country, where the technology boom began earlier than in the populous northern states, three (Maharashtra, Andra Pradesh, and Karnatka) are probably just above the replacement rate, and two (Tamil Nadu and Kerala) are already below the replacement rate.

China. Before 9/11 it was not Islamist terrorism that was regarded as the greatest long-term threat or competitor to American views and values. That honor went to the 1.3 billion Chinese, projected to grow to 1.5 billion before beginning a decline. As already noted, the Chinese economic story has been remarkable. Such economic progress under free-market principles is all to the good. America is not hurt by other nations growing richer under market systems. But China has by no means matched its free-market economics with a move toward political liberty.

One day China may be free in the full sense of the word. Some small movement in that direction now appears to be taking place. Ezra Vogel, former director of Harvard's Fairbank Center for East Asian Research, writes that China's opening and reform may be yielding "an intellectual vitality that may be as broad and deep as the Western Renaissance." He cites the broad activity going on at Harvard and many other large universities, and notes that an increasing number of Chinese graduates are now returning to China. The courses of study include engineering, science, medicine, law (including the study of comparative democracy), health, business, design (China has more ongoing construction projects than any nation in the world), and city planning. Members of the People's Liberation Army study international security. The Chinese Communist Central Party

School invites American faculty to lecture to midcareer officials in China, in part to talk about democratic governance.*

This is a potentially great story which could shape the future. But for now China cannot yet be counted on the side of those forces in the world that seek to expand human liberty. As the saying goes, "Rubber bends, plastic breaks." Democratic flexibility provides the malleability and lubrication necessary to settle internal problems without tanks and without slaughter. Its historical record is impressive. Such a democratic political system has not yet been instituted in China. An internal Chinese crack-up could lead to a global disaster.

Because of a large population and growing income, China has been able to create the world's second most powerful military force. It is a nuclear power with an estimated 400 to 450 nuclear warheads (strategic and tactical). While its military forces have been reduced somewhat—to about 2 million men on active duty and another 1.5 million in the reserve militia—China's troop strength is the largest in the world, including that of the United States.

Chinese foreign policy has been seen as hostile to the interests of the West. Moreover, its important neighbors are constantly afraid that China might turn expansionist. (The Chinese have occupied Tibet.) Either by treaty or by informal arrangement, many of China's neighbors—including Japan and South Korea—are defended by American military power, made possible in part by our own large and growing population and high income. It is not inconceivable that one day some of those brilliant Western-educated Chinese students will be using their talents in the service of a China that is an American adversary. That would be a global tragedy of the first magnitude.

Islam, and terrorism. And then there are the Islamist terrorists, who are now in clear first place as global villains. There are somewhat more than a billion Muslims in the world. Arabs are a subset, making up about a quarter of that number. Freedom House rates the Arab nations as the most repressive in the world.

But even there, some muffled bells of freedom can be heard. Meetings held by the UN Development Programme have gathered Arab intellectuals who have called for "promoting open intellectual inquiry."

Washington Post, December 5, 2003.

The UN-published document (the "Arab Human Development Report") highlights the following statement by Abdul Rahman al-Kawakibi: "We have become accustomed to regarding abject submission as polite deference; obsequiousness as courtesy; sycophancy as oratory; bombast as substance; the acceptance of humiliation as modesty; the acceptance of injustice as obedience; and the pursuit of human entitlements as arrogance. Our inverted system portrays the pursuit of the simplest knowledge as presumption; aspirations for the future as impossible dreams; courage as overreaching audacity; inspiration as folly; chivalry as aggression; free speech as insolence and free thinking as heresy."

Demographically, the document says, "the emigration of qualified Arabs constitutes a form of reverse development aid." Under the heading of "The Arab Brain Drain," it notes that "Roughly 25 percent of first degree graduates from Arab universities in 1995/96 emigrated. Between 1998 and 2000 more than 15,000 Arab doctors migrated." The document declares a "freedom deficit."

In all, Muslims make up about one in six human beings on the planet. Their numbers are still growing, but, as noted earlier, their fertility rate is falling, in some places rapidly. Indonesia is the most populous Muslim nation in the world with 212 million people. Its TFR has fallen from 5.7 children per woman in 1955–1960 to 2.35 in 2000–2005, which is just about .1 of a child higher than the replacement rate when calculated for an LDC. It seems pretty clear that Indonesia's TFR will drop below the replacement rate soon, and then, as the calendar moves forward, toward the UN's new 1.85 number, and perhaps below that. Still, because of the powerful forces of demographic momentum, Indonesia's population is projected to grow to 294 million people by midcentury before beginning a demographic decline.

Most Muslim nations are experiencing a continuing drop in fertility and rising populations, which will begin falling toward midcentury. Give or take a couple of hundred million, Muslims should remain about one-sixth of the global population. The threat from Muslims is not demographic.

The Muslim population in the world is composed mostly of poor people. Remember our concept that warmaking capacity requires numbers plus wealth. That pretty well rules out a traditional cross-border military threat by Muslims to any well-to-do armed modern nation. But it does not rule out direct warfare with other poor nations. In recent years, whenever Muslim countries have been in close proximity to non-Muslim countries, violent conflict has emerged.

It should go without saying that the vast majority of Muslims are peace-loving people, seeking a good life for themselves and their families. Many have combined their Muslim faith with a modernist value system. Many Muslims are governed by some form of democratic rule, and while such democratic development is usually in its infancy, it seems to be growing. (But there are no Arab democracies.)

As shown by the example of fertility rates, we live in one world. Fertility fell first among the Western nations, now it is declining most everywhere. Mass democracy in the modern age began in America. As the data shown earlier reveal, such governance is now spreading globally. It will reach the Arab world, sooner or later.

At times during his presidential campaign of 2000, Governor George W. Bush said things that some observers thought sounded a bit isolationist (a complex term). Bush suggested in many speeches that America should be more "humble" in its dealings with other nations (pronounced "umble" in Texas). He said American troops should not be used for "nation-building." In the long-running argument between the American "realists" and American "idealists," he seemed to come down on the side of the realists. (Those too have always been terms more complex than the labels made them out to be.)

Then something changed. One may surmise that the troubles in the war in Iraq had at least something to do with it. As this book is written, I do not know how that war will turn out. Its proximate cause was to rid a gruesome tyrant of biological, chemical, and nuclear weapons of mass destruction. Many months after the American soldiers won the military part of the war, the WMDs were still not found. There was an apparent massive intelligence failure, not only by America but by other nations as well. The death of many American servicemen and Iraqi civilians during the insurgencies in 2004 were heartrending. Abuse of Iraqi prisoners and the subsequent media firestorm shamed Americans. The ghastly murders of American civilians by Iraqis was outrageous. International public opinion was against the war from the start, and declined from there.*

Parallels have been drawn to Vietnam and an Iraqi "quagmire." I am dubious. Both President Bush and putative Democratic presidential candidate John Kerry have pledged not to "cut and run." We shall see about that. The important thing to remember is that America recovered from Vietnam, and in not such a long time. All the things described in this book happened notwithstanding Vietnam, including very specifically the global growth of liberty described here.

Wars, like life, can be about several things at once. Like most good salesmen, President Bush had more than one item in his kit bag. After the Iraq situation began turning sour, he started emphasizing how important it would be for America to bring democracy to the Middle East, and Iraq would be the true test. Some of his strong views are excerpted below. I don't believe that Iraq will become a model of democracy and liberty overnight. It is likely to be a mess for a long time. But by my lights, if Iraq moves only very partially toward some sort of pluralistic democratic governance, the war will have been worth it, notwithstanding the tragic loss of life. And it is no accident that rather suddenly the talk about democracy has reverberated throughout the Arab world.

In a series of three major speeches in 2003, Bush began making his case that democracy is America's mission. The venues were the National Endowment for Democracy, Buckingham Palace, and the American Enterprise Institute. They are worth extended quotation.

I mix and match from the three speeches:

"In the early 1970s there were about 40 democracies in the world. . . . As the twentieth century ended there were around 120 democracies. . . . Seventy-four years ago, the London *Times* declared nine-tenths of the population of India to be 'illiterates not caring a fig for politics.' Yet when Indian democracy was imperiled in the 1970s, the Indian people showed their commitment to liberty in a national ref-

---

*Ivan Kratsev of Bulgaria's Center for Liberal Strategies maintains that the twenty-first century may come to be known as the "anti-American Century," a view that seems premature.

erendum that saved their form of government. . . . [China now has] a sliver, a fragment of liberty. Yet China's people will eventually want their liberty pure and whole. . . . Eventually men and women who are allowed to control their own wealth will insist on controlling their own lives and their own country. . . . In many Middle Eastern countries poverty is deep and is spreading; women lack rights, and are denied schooling. Whole societies remain stagnant while the world moves ahead. These are not failures of a culture or a religion. These are failures of political and economic doctrines."

"Successful societies limit the power of the state and the power of the military . . . protect freedom . . . respond to the will of the people . . . protect freedom with consistent and impartial rule of law . . . allow room for healthy civic institutions, for political parties and labor unions and independent newspapers and broadcast media . . . guarantee religious liberty, the right to serve God and honor God without fear of persecution. . . . [They] privatize their economies and secure the rights of property. They prohibit and punish official corruption and invest in the health and education of their people. And instead of directing hatred and resentment against others, successful societies appeal to the hopes of their own people. . . . Freedom can be the future of every nation. . . . The advance of freedom leads to peace. . . . With all of these tests and all the challenges of our age, this is, above all, the age of liberty."

"These terrorists target the innocent, and they kill by the thousands. And they would, if they gain the weapons they seek, kill by the millions and not be finished. The greatest threat of our age is nuclear, chemical, or biological weapons in the hands of terrorists and the dictators who aid them. The evil is in plain sight. The danger only increases with denial. Great responsibilities fall once again to the great democracies. We will face these threats with open eyes, and we will defeat them."

"[America] is committed to this great democratic alliance [NATO] and believes it must have the will and the capacity to act beyond Europe when threats emerge. [Security comes about from] our commitment to the global expansion of democracy. . . . Lasting peace is gained as justice and democracy advance. . . . In our conflict with terror and tyranny, we have an unmatched advantage, a power that cannot be resisted, and that is the appeal of freedom to all mankind. . . . Freedom, by definition, must be chosen, and defended by those who choose it. . . . Our part, as free nations, is to ally ourselves with reform, wherever it occurs. . . . No longer should we think of tyranny because it is temporarily convenient. Tyranny is never benign to its victims, and our great democracies should oppose tyranny wherever it is found.

"The world has a clear interest in the spread of democratic values, because stable and free nations do not breed the ideologies of murder. . . . [The United Nations] was created, as Winston Churchill said, to 'make sure that the force of right will . . . be protected by the right of force. . . . We go forward with confidence, because we trust in the power of human freedom to change lives and nations. By the resolve and purpose of America, and our friends and allies, we will make this an age of progress and liberty. Free people will set the course of history, and free people will keep the peace in the world."

The words fill many Americans with spirit. But at the moment many people around the world do not like the United States, making American leadership of the cause of liberty more difficult. A survey in March 2004 by Harris Interactive yielded this conclusion: "When people in the five largest European countries think of the United States, they tend, on balance, to feel positively about the American people, American films and television programs, the quality of life in America, and how Americans do business. On the other hand, large majorities of Europeans have negative opinions of President Bush, U.S. policies in Iraq and Afghanistan, and recent American foreign policy." It is fair to say that such sentiments are shared in most parts of the world.

President Bush's words are not humble thoughts. In early 2000, during the primary campaigns, I traveled for two days with Senator John McCain on his "Straight Talk Express" through the snows of New Hampshire. At each stop his most popular line was, "We have to believe in something bigger than ourselves." Those Bush speeches express mine. The purveying of liberty is the province not only of Freedom House, neo-conservatives, the *Wall Street Journal*, and human rights organizations. It is now the stated, and restated, policy of the government of the United States.

I am a great admirer of the late Senator Henry M. ("Scoop") Jackson, on whose behalf I worked during his presidential campaigns of 1972 and 1976. Upon reflection, Scoop's greatest contribution to American geopolitical life may well have been the "Jackson-Vanik Amendment," dealing with the right of Jews, Pentecostals, and others to emigrate from the Soviet Union in return for the Soviets gaining "Most Favored Nation" trading status. In so doing he linked individual liberty with international policy, no small matter.

What we are going through now has been described by Eliot Cohen of the Center for Strategic and International Studies as "World War Four." One and Two occurred in the first part of the last century. The cold war was Three. The terror attacks on America and elsewhere constitute Four. It seems like an appropriate classification. The terror is worldwide and has wrought great havoc. It will almost surely last for a long time.

The sworn enemy of Al-Qaeda is precisely what we in Western civilization stand for and what we are dedicated to promulgating further: modernism, Westernism, liberty, Americanism, call it what it you will. To Osama bin Laden and his ancillary attack organizations, the enemy has been the people and symbols of Western civilization. What we find to be the most successful moment in history, the terrorists see as the indicia of blasphemy. Where we glory in the ongoing spread of human liberty, they see the enemy. Where we see modernism as ongoing progress, they fear such progress.

The terrorist threat presents an extremely difficult situation for America and for the nations of the West. Except for America, these nations are on a path to population decline of major proportions. And because the population of working-age people yields wealth, with each passing year Westerners will be living with a smaller proportion of global wealth. Although the wealth gap is still very large, and will remain so for a very long time, that is the trend. (Some LDCs—South Korea and Taiwan, for example—have already graduated to modern income standards.)

These numbers suggest several alternative strategies for the nations of the West. The first is some form of mild semi-isolationism, that is, of doing nothing new or assertive, or very little. That seemed to be an aspect of the position that Bush laid out in his 2000 campaign. The nations and peoples of the West—that is, America, Europe, and Japan—over a period of time could in effect say, "We have no grand goal." Trade and the normal intercourse of nations would of course continue. We would continue to try to combat terrorism because we must. The West is still so much more powerful and so much wealthier than the nations of the non-Western world that there would be no short-term direct threat to our well-being, with the possible exception of the terrorists. But, it is said, terrorism is the weapon of the weak. They can scare us, and they have, but they won't destroy us. We would support liberty, but it would not be high on the agenda.

The second option has been laid out earlier but now deserves fuller attention. Most of us Westerners believe that what has been created in the West is the best way of life yet seen. Its hallmark is the defense and extension of human liberty. A strong case can be made that the modernism that brought us human liberty has brought the human species to its most successful moment. But it may not continue. None of us can divine the future. Civilizations rise and fall. Many historians believe that Hitler's Nazis could have won World War II if he had not made some major blunders. He came very close to routing the Soviets. Churchill and the English stood strong much against the prevailing odds. The Americans lost much of their fleet at Pearl Harbor. Finally America and its Allies, including the Soviets, turned the tide against the Nazis, the Japanese, and assorted other states that thought totalitarianism was a pretty good idea. It was a close call. It is fair to say that if the totalitarian powers led by Germany and Japan had prevailed, we would not be having this conversation about the global extension of human liberty today.

The cold war too could have been lost. In Marxism the Soviets had a seductive socialist global ideology that appealed to many nations and many people over many years. They conquered nations and ruled others through somewhat less direct force. In actual combat situations the Communists did very well. They fought to a draw in Korea. Their attempted movement of missiles into Cuba in 1963 seemed like a standoff, but the Soviets probably prevailed: they got the Americans to remove their missiles in Turkey because of their Cuban threat. The Communists won in Vietnam. A strong peace movement in Europe diminished European military strength. The cold war too could have gone the other way. Had it, we would not be concerned about the global extension of human liberty today.

The point is elemental: we don't know what comes next. Under both Democratic and Republican administrations, the United States has prospered in recent decades, as the data here has shown. The movement toward social and economic liberty is flourishing. Ever since I have been able to read, I have noted keen observers who have said, "The world is at a turning point," or some variant thereof. This is not to say they were wrong. But neither does it mean that the world is not now at a pivotal moment. I believe it is.

This may be the unique moment to steer mankind toward Churchill's uplands. What we do now will likely affect the course of mankind for decades and centuries. It is a propitious moment. We should not forget that, notwithstanding the ongoing threat from global terror, the fall of the Soviet Union left us without a full-bodied enemy.

Senator Daniel P. Moynihan probably contributed more powerful political phrases than any man in recent times. He had a beauty for the prospect we now consider: the Liberty party. Moynihan believed that if the freedom-lovers of the world, and the freedom-loving nations of the world, could come together in a serious and structured way, we could make history of a monumental sort. The idea has some demographic implications: the numbers of people in the nations that currently make up Western civilization are going way down proportional to the rest of the world. In that sense we Westerners are starting off behind and will be falling further behind. Fertility rates far below replacement levels may be linked to modernity and personal liberty, but by definition they cannot be sustained in the long term.

A "party" or a "movement" can do things that individual nations cannot do alone, no matter how passionate they may be. For example, NATO would not let Spain and Portugal join their club until the dictators Franco and Salazar had passed on and those nations became legitimate democracies. And, of course, the Eastern European nations could not join the democratic club until the dismemberment of the Soviet Union.

Many of the great movements in human history have occurred because of—movements. It is time that the cause of human freedom and liberty be treated as a movement, not just as a splendid idea.

Socialism was a vastly successful movement and party for a century and more. Some of its ideas remain, though often as features of social democracy. At one point the majority of the people in the world lived in nations that subscribed to the socialist ideal. There was a "Socialist Internationale" that attempted to coordinate policies for the true believers. It represented a movement. The Comintern in a more top-down manner, performed much the same role for the Communists.*

Not much in human history has been accomplished when the players are halfhearted in their beliefs. I would wager we will have plenty of halfheartedness toward the geopolitical idea of putting the defense and extension of human liberty high on our agenda. It won't happen unless we believe in it deeply and teach it to our children.

Surely every nation has priorities it seeks to pursue. Every nation has an international economic agenda concerning trade and economic growth. Such interests will continue, as well they must. Within nations, political parties will argue about regulation and taxes. Ever thus. The most important aspect of a Liberty party is that its members believe it to be great and grand, superseding the day-to-day work of politics.

If there is to be a Liberty party, it should at least have an office. There was meeting of "the community of only free nations" in Warsaw in June 2000, and a similar gathering in Seoul in 2002. Another meeting is scheduled for Santiago in 2005. But this "movement" doesn't even have a hole-in-the-wall office! If we are to take this seriously, let's have an office. The columnist Jonathan Rauch writes that one day a "Community of Democracies" will compete with the UN, or become its successor.

The National Endowment for Democracy is America's keystone agency for promoting democratic values. It was established in 1983 amidst much controversy in Congress. The original NED budget was $18 million per year. Now it is officially $40 million, and President Bush has asked for a doubling of that amount, with the new monies slated for the Greater Middle East, from Morocco to Pakistan.

But as NED president Carl Gershman notes, the $40 million figure is greatly understated. The Agency for International Development

*See Joshua Muravchik's *Heaven on Earth: The Rise and Fall of Socialism* (San Francisco, 2003).

and the Department of State both contribute funds, as do other institutions. In all, one estimate has it that the United States spends more than $600 million per year on promoting democracy, about a quarter of which goes directly through NED and its Republican, Democratic, labor, and business institutes. Like others in the democracy movement, Gershman stresses that democracy can only be encouraged, not imposed. About five hundred grants go out each year to Non-Governmental Organizations for a variety of democracy projects. Building democracy is retail work as well as wholesale, he says. It is an idea whose time has come.

Nor is Congress a problem any longer. In 2003, by unanimous vote in the Senate and by 390 to 1 in the House, a resolution was passed congratulating NED on the occasion of its twenty years of operation. The agency has also played an important role in encouraging the creation of NED-like groups elsewhere in the free world. They exist now in the UK, Canada, Spain, Sweden, Norway, the Netherlands, France, Poland, Taiwan, Australia, and the European Union. Other nations are getting ready to participate.

Because the LDCs are growing rapidly, America should give them more promotion-of-freedom aid directly and through multi-national organizations. In repressive countries we should do more to publicize groups and people seeking to democratize their governments. We should put governmental pressure on governments that repress those who hoist the flag of democracy. We should encourage, and pay for, freedom activists to visit America. As Fareed Zakaria has written, there is much more to democracy than just having an election. Some countries have had elections featuring one man, one vote, one time.

From 1953 to 1999 the United States Information Agency helped "tell America's story to the world." But the heist of funds from the USIA in 1999 was craven and foolhardy. The team of Jesse Helms, chairman of the Senate Foreign Relations Committee, and the Clinton foreign policy apparatus headed by Secretary of State Madeline Albright, "subsumed" the USIA. Its budget was raped, and former USIA officers, who brought credibility to what could have been viewed as straight propaganda, now are middle level public affairs officers. Both are needed.

Notwithstanding the misfortune of the USIA, America still has a wide array of tools for what is called "public diplomacy." These include the Voice of America, broadcasting forty-four languages, Radio Free Europe/Radio Liberty in twenty-seven languages, and Radio Free Asia in nine languages. To this aggregation something new has been added: the Middle East Television Network, which broadcasts Arab-language television via Alhurra, and an Arab-language pop radio channel, Radio Sawa, heavily skewed to music. How effective this programming will be remains to be seen, aimed as it is at a part of the world where America is particularly unpopular and regularly reviled by the Arabic satellite news television channel Al Jazeera and others. But now we are trying.

After 9/11 one popular question was "Why do they hate us?" One speculative answer concerned the idea that the "sole super-power" will always be disliked and distrusted. Perhaps so. But it is a strange situation in a world where ten million people fill out lottery forms to try to get a relatively few slots for legal immigration to America, and a world where so many people everywhere have aped American views and values. Right now, mostly keyed to the Iraq war, global views about America are particularly low. What should America do? My view, sketched out earlier in this chapter, is to continue to pursue our missions. America still has a great story to tell.

The Liberty movement won't be smooth sailing; Samuel Huntington writes of "reverse waves." Democracy has moved forward, then faltered. The path has been ascendant, but bad things can happen in good countries. That democracy is growing now doesn't mean there will not be setbacks.

Recently there has been much written and much spoken about the idea of an "American Empire." Should America be an empire? Can America be effective as an imperium?

The intent of this chapter is that America constitutes an empire of ideals, and should be such an empire. The core idea is a noble one, concerning individual liberty in more places, for more people. Writing in May of 2004, Fouad Ajami pointed out that there are times when America is its own worst enemy, and that the self-flagellation over the events in Iraq was one such time. It is hard to avoid that in a free country in an election year. But we can try harder, and we should.

CHAPTER TWELVE

Is There an Immigration Solution?

RICH COUNTRIES are losing people and are concerned about it, for good reason. Poor countries are growing substantially, albeit at much slower rates than expected, and they regard population growth as a liability, at least temporarily. It takes no giant policy theoretician to say, Why don't we move some of the "extra" Third Worlders to the emptying lands of the First World? It would also make sense in terms of age distribution for the receiving nations. Immigration typically yields "instant adults" who pay taxes.

For an example, consider the situation in United States as calculated in the late 1990s. With somewhat different numbers plugged in, it would be relevant today for most of the other modern nations in the world. As mentioned earlier, the median age of an immigrant to America was twenty-eight. These were men and women who had been raised and educated on someone else's national and parental budgets, saving monies for American taxpayers. Once an immigrant arrives in America, he or she will then pay into Social Security and Medicare for about forty to forty-five years before drawing any benefits. Ongoing immigration to America would thus cut about 28 percent off the projected Social Security shortfall. And immigrants do not add to certain major fixed costs of the federal government, like national defense or the existing interest on the national debt.

Dueling economic studies debate whether immigration helps or harms the American economy. "The New Americans," prepared by the National Research Council (1997), shows that immigration is generally good for the American public economy. It also disaggregates the value of the governmental economic benefits of immigration. A typical immigrant pays in $80,000 (net) more in taxes than he or she receives in government services over the course of a lifetime. (State governments lose $25,000 while the federal government gains $105,000.) If we took in more immigrants, there would be greater per capita federal receipts and somewhat less of a Social Security crisis.

Other studies, particularly the work of George Borjas of Harvard, come to different, mildly negative conclusions. But all this involves comparatively small money over the course of a lifetime, one way or the other.

I have testified before Congress several times on this issue, and I have seen its members appear stunned that a growing America has vast domestic and geopolitical implications. Most American legislators have not thought through what the world would be like if America were not a big, growing country. They hone in on the next election quite well, however.

True, immigration invariably comes with problems. The "settler nations"—America, Canada, and Australia—are growing and generally prospering. But even in these nations immigration increases the stress quotient. For example, many Americans, particularly in California, fear the "Mexifornication" of their state, if not the entire nation. A few Australians still pine for the old "white only" immigration policy. Some Canadians don't like the idea that the Province of Quebec has an independent immigration policy tilted to French-speakers from all over the world, who demand, and get, bilingual signs throughout Canada.

Nor is America immune to anti-immigrant sentiment, as noted earlier. In June 2001, Gallup asked respondents, "In your view, should immigration be kept at its present level, increased, or decreased?" Results: 42 percent "about right," 14 percent "more," 41 percent "less." After 9/11, in June 2003, the numbers were different, but not massively so: 37 percent "about right," 13 percent "more," and 47 percent "less." In either case, Americans were not marching in the streets calling for more immigrants. Good comparative international data is not readily available, but it is fair to say that no country is now looking for Arab or Muslim immigrants.

After 9/11, America and the world had good reason to fear Arab and Muslim immigration. President Bush invited groups of Arabs and Muslims to the White House to explain to the public that Islam is a religion of love, and that the 9/11 bombers were a small minority of extremists. He would not have been a very good president if he said anything else. Still, the terrorists were Arabs.

And America is a happy party compared to other areas. The anti-Muslim feeling in Europe was marked before 9/11. (Most European immigrants come from Arab North Africa. This was once viewed as primarily a French problem, except for Germany, where the distaste was expressed at Turks.) After 9/11, anti-Muslim sentiment grew more intense everywhere in Europe, and elsewhere for that matter.

The Japanese anti-immigrant sentiment is, if anything, worse than the European. UN data show the Japanese annual immigration rate at .4 of a person per thousand people, compared to .9 for Europe and 4.1 for the United States. (Many Japanese believe that the foreigners have a bad odor.)

The American immigration problem is mild by European or Japanese standards. Immigrants and their descendants live bunched up or dispersed, as they choose—more and more dispersed as the generations roll on. Many Korean Americans in Southern California live in "Koreatown." Many Cuban Americans live in or around "Little Havana" in Miami. Large communities of Mexican Americans reside in many places. Many Chinese Americans live in or around the "Chinatowns" that are found in many major American cities. Many Arab Americans live in the vicinity of Dearborn, Michigan, near Detroit. During presidential election years, you will find candidates for president and vice president showing up in the Dearborn area to let Arab Americans know how valued they are as part of the great American mosaic. (Michigan is a "swing state.")

Not very many immigrants in Europe become citizens, and few vote. The French Chamber of Deputies does not have even one member of Arab or Muslim ancestry.* And virtually none attend the

---

*Imagine the U.S. House of Representatives without black Members!

grandes écoles that lead to access in the French elite, according to an article by Reihan Salam in the New Republic Online. Salam maintains that such discriminatory policy has encouraged the virulently anti-Semitic and separatist French Muslim party.

In his book *The New Americans*, Michael Barone counts blacks as "immigrants." Like many immigrants—but usually more so—most African Americans live in neighborhoods where they are the majority or the totality of the population.* But they have substantially more contact with other Americans than they used to, in the workplace and in the upper grades of school. In the 1970s Whitney Young, then president of the Urban League, told my co-author Richard Scammon and me a story about Martin Luther King: "Martin told me: never forget, blacks in America are materialistic, religious, and patriotic." On the whole I believe that is still a valid general description, albeit with some violent tragedy mixed in.

Moreover, there is substantial intermarriage going on, less among blacks but growing quite rapidly, and well over half among some other immigrant groups. Soon it will be hard to tell the players without a scorecard. In the decades to come, intermarriage may solve many of America's problems while in some cases causing personal anguish among parents and grandparents.

Immigration comes in two segments: high skilled and low skilled. The high-skilled group is important for a country seeking to produce high added-value goods and services in order to maintain a growing standard of living. Such countries, like Canada and Germany, frequently offer inducements to new immigrants. It is a good idea, though the American Congress has done very little in this regard, preferring to give immigration slots to relatives of families already here, and lesser amounts to workers needed by business. The Canadians have instituted a rather sophisticated "point system" designed to bring high-quality immigrants to the country. (Canada's annual immigration rate is 4.9 persons per thousand per year, somewhat higher than the

---

*Don't believe the word "segregation" when used in this context, or in the context of school populations or the workplace. Segregation was a *law* that prohibited blacks from going to school with whites or living in certain neighborhoods, etc. Segregation is now *against the law*.

4.1 of the United States.) Seven Canadian immigrants to the United States have won Nobel Prizes. Go south, young man!

More important, and less recognized, is the need for low-skill immigrants in the modern nations. More than a need, it will be a necessity. With aging populations, the demand for senior care services will be enormous. Who will staff the low-skill hospital jobs? Who will do the 24/7 home nursing? In wealthy societies, who will mow the lawns, clean the houses, deliver the pizza, and serve as chambermaids in the hotels? In most well-to-do countries those jobs are performed by immigrants and their offspring while upward mobility proceeds, albeit sometimes quite slowly. There will not be many responses from Americans for a help-wanted advertisement to scrub toilet bowls.

Talk to cab drivers in major cities in America and you will often be informed that the driver is sending money home every month to his aged parent, or to send a younger sibling to school. This is voluntary person-to-person money. In some countries, including Albania, El Salvador, Jamaica, Jordan, Nicaragua, and Yemen, such payments make up more than 10 percent of the Gross Domestic Product. Remittances are Mexico's third-largest source of national income. They also provide investment funds for entrepreneurs. As noted, such payments are generally immune from the corruption that is apparently endemic when foreign aid goes from rich governments to poor governments or through international institutions.

The UN's first global immigration report in 2002 noted that the number of immigrants globally was at an all-time high of about 175 million people. The United States, with 35 million immigrants, had the highest total number. Russia was in second place with 13 million immigrants (many of them Russians returning from the former Soviet republics), and Germany in third place with 7 million. In the 1990–2000 decade alone, the number of immigrants in the world grew by 14 percent. Including the children of immigrants, the five leading nations are the United Arab Emirates (74 percent), Kuwait (58 percent), Jordan (40 percent), Israel (37 percent), and Singapore (34 percent).

While there are more immigrants than ever, there are nowhere near enough to deal with the massive structural magnitude of the problems at hand. A total of 3 percent of the global population are immigrants, but that amount, sliced and diced as you please, would not come close to providing substantial help for the looming pension shortfall in Europe. And despite the fact that scores of millions of ambitious people are ready to emigrate to places with a higher standard of living, even if it involves a high degree of danger, many of those places dislike newcomers. In a tough game, I think the immigrants will win. Someone has to empty those bedpans. And sooner or later (probably later), Europeans will have to learn how to accommodate pluralism. (Historian Jeffrey Williamson of Harvard believes that immigration will rise, not fall, as peoples in the LDCs gain access to more money; the act of immigration with its attendant costs of travel, he says, will be easier. Perhaps so. But over the medium term, as populations sink because of dramatically falling TFRs, that is not likely to happen. The available pool of immigrants will also fall.)

UNTIL 9/11, one could imagine an evolutionary process whereby immigration could solve some of the foreseeable global problems. But what happened on 9/11, and afterward, has changed a great deal. It is one thing to be pro-immigration (like me) and say don't worry, it will all work out. It becomes an entirely different matter when immigrants or foreigners fly airplanes into the Pentagon and the World Trade Center. If the terrorists can scare a population into severely restricting immigration, they will have accomplished a mighty deed.

Still, even reducing immigration to the United States was a near impossible task, even before 9/11. One late afternoon, as dusk was settling between California and Baja, I sat in a Jeep with a Border Patrol officer (a Mexican American) and watched as posses formed on the Mexican side of the fence. Small bonfires sprung alight as the leaders briefed their human customers.

Some immigrants would make it across the border, scampering across U.S. Route 8, near San Diego. Others would be caught and sent back to Mexico, from where most would try again. A few years ago Pat Buchanan's idea of a fence to keep Mexican illegals out of the United States drew withering comments. It doesn't sound so tough now that the Israelis are using it as a potential remedy against terrorism.

Illegal immigration has proved to be about as close to an insoluble policy problem as exists in modern societies. Two general scenarios have emerged. Some Americans seek to reduce massive amounts of legal immigration, with an emphasis on Arabs or Muslims. The Europeans are more forthright about these matters: they have been singling out Arabs and Muslims as immigrants they don't want and in some cases seeking to expel some of those they have.

A new immigration stream is now forming from Latin America to Europe. From a European perspective, the new Latin immigrants work hard, at low wages, at the worst jobs, and are not seen as potential terrorists. Indeed, that may be the sort of global immigration solution that emerges: rich countries taking in needed immigrants from poor Latin American, sub-Saharan, and non-Muslim Asian countries while Muslims seeking a better life suffer from the actions of Muslim terrorists.

And then there is the case of South Korea, one of the important sources of immigrants for the United States. But these days South Korea is also *receiving* immigrants, South Koreans who are returning and others. More LDCs will be following that trend as economic conditions improve more rapidly there than in the modern nations.

I HAVE DESCRIBED why I believe immigration has been good for America and the world, and will be good for America and the world in the intermediate term, out to 2050. Now let us look a long way out.

Imagine you are an American in the Census year of 1800. You have 5.3 million fellow Americans; let us call it a flat 5 million. And some fellow with a slide rule comes along and tells you that in the next 200 years the American population will grow to 280 million people. Be serious, you tell him. He persists and says that by 2050 the U.S. population will be 400 million people, the richest, freest, and most powerful nation the world has ever seen.

These sorts of things do happen in demographics. In the UN "Medium" scenario for the year 2300—way out—India's population will be 1.372 billion and China's 1.285 billion. And the little United States will still be in third place with 493 million people, up another hundred million people from 2050 but still well less than half of the billionaires. In short, America is a big country, growing bigger, but not anywhere near the biggest.

It is hard to imagine it right now, but as world population sinks, as it will, a person (read, immigrant) becomes more valuable. (Supply and demand again.) People produce wealth. More people produce more wealth. More people produce more power. If you're selling something, like the promotion and extension of liberty, you have a better hand to play when you have more people. (It also helps to have a great idea.)

Area used to be an important indicator of national strength. For the record, America and China have roughly the same area, about 3.6 million square miles. India has an area about a third the size of America or China. Russia is the world's largest nation with an area of more than twice that of America or China. Area doesn't matter much any more; neither does that old standby "arable land." There is plenty of food for a healthy diet for the people of Earth.

According to the U.S. Census Bureau, in 2002–2003 America took in about 1.5 million immigrants, legal and illegal. Some experts think the number may be a little on the low side. From that one may subtract about 200,000 Americans who emigrate. While immigrants from Latin America make up the largest *number*, in recent years the most rapid *rate* of immigration is among Asians, the so-called "model minority." Next to Spanish, the language most likely to be spoken at home is Chinese.

When I mention this, the first question people ask is usually: But where would they live? The answer has been noted earlier: most anywhere. In the suburbs, for one. The American housing market has been a wonder to behold (in 1910 just 12 percent of Americans lived in suburbs, that is, near but not in a big city, and in 2000 the rate was 52 percent). Cities themselves have been rejuvenated by immigrants— by Dominicans in New York City and Vietnamese in the Orange County and Pasadena areas of southern California. In the midcontinent are areas that are growing only slowly (and sometimes losing absolute numbers of people) and are fully habitable, albeit typically with older populations. These communities already have streets, schools, sewers, and the infrastructure needed for a thriving community—and low crime rates too. Some rural areas have emptied out; in 1900 it took thirty-eight hours of agricultural labor to cultivate an acre of corn, in 1997 just two. The worst sections of some inner-cities have lost people for many reasons, principally crime.

I am also asked, Where will the additional Americans work? Where will the jobs come from? The answer is: mostly from creative Americans, building better mousetraps or creating new biotech medicines, in the private sector. In the 1990s the states with the fastest-growing immigrant populations were North Carolina (274 percent), Georgia (233 percent), Nevada (202 percent), Arkansas (196 percent), and Utah (171 percent). As noted several times earlier in this volume, the wealth-producing jobs will not typically come from government.

America has an excellent track record in helping immigrants become productive people. I live in Washington, D.C. When I take a cab and the driver's accent is foreign, which it typically is, I make it a point to try to strike up a conversation. I ask him where he is from. He tells me. I then ask, "How do you like America?" The answer I get, in one variant or another, is almost always on this theme: "There is great opportunity here, but you have to work very hard." Typically there are no limitations on the hours a cab driver can work. It is a hard way to make a living, though with long hours the income can be good. Other immigrants find better, higher-paid, or easier occupations. And others do work that may be unappealing to many Americans—plucking chickens, picking fruit, working as chambermaids, taking care of children as nannies.

In principle, I do not believe the proposals for an "amnesty" for illegal immigrants are salutary. America did that in 1986. I was in favor of it then—as a one-time shot. But now new proposals are afoot to legalize illegals one more time. The new proposals are sponsored by President Bush and a number of legislators from both parties. All deny their programs are an "amnesty," but in essence they are. The logical effect of such legislation will be to encourage still more illegality. The message to potential illegal immigrants is clear: Come in illegally, wait a few years, and get legalized, at least for a few years.

An amnesty program, by whatever name, is not voter friendly. In the California Recall Circus of 2003, the proposed policy change was to make illegal* entry even easier by granting driving licences to

*We have a wonderful way with euphemisms. In this situation we have moved from "illegal" to "undocumented" and now sometimes to "unauthorized."

persons with no valid proof of legal residence in the United States. Both Lieutenant Governor Cruz Bustamante and the hounded Governor Gray Davis came out in favor of granting such "legal" drivers licenses. Governor Arnold Schwarzenegger (an immigrant) opposed them—and won the election.

I don't like amnesty, but upon painful reflection, I think it should be done. First, there is not much to do about it; illegals get in whether we like it or not. But we should remember that they are for the most part people with some gumption. The word on the street is that they work hard. It is not an easy choice to leave home for a dangerous journey and an inhospitable welcome.

The Urban Institute estimates there are 9.3 million illegal immigrants in America, representing 26 percent of the total foreign-born population. Mexicans make up more than half the illegals (5.3 million people). The reason for Mexican preponderance is elemental: the 2,500-mile-long common border with the United States. It is easier to come into America illegally from Mexico than it is from Indonesia. As great a country as America is, we cannot move the border. About 2.2 million illegals (23 percent) hail from other Latin American countries. Thus about three-quarters the illegals are from Latin America. The results of the 2000 U.S. Census show that about half a million illegal immigrants come to America each year. (Earlier estimates from the Census Bureau were in the 200,000 to 300,000 range. The anti-immigration hard-liners were right on this one.)

In all, illegal immigrants make up about 3 percent of the U.S. population. That is a significant amount but a very long way from overwhelming.

The illegals present a major social problem for America because they live "in the shadows." An estimated 15 to 17 percent of illegals are children. They have typically grown up in America. They seek upward mobility. Most finish high school. Many want to go on to community college, junior college, or higher. Their illegality can make it difficult to get into schools of higher education, or, if they do, to get in-state tuition or financial aid.

Who is helped by that? Their illegality inhibits their geographical mobility, eliminating a classic way that Americans upgrade their economic standing. Illegals often cannot get health insurance. The new welfare laws make it difficult for them to get "the helping hand" (temporarily, while looking for a job). They have difficulty enrolling in government-sponsored English-language courses. They can't vote. It is difficult for them to participate in their communities. Their illegality makes it harder for police to do their work if the illegals are of a criminal bent.

The Manhattan Institute's Tamar Jacoby, editor and co-author of *Reinventing the Melting Pot*, makes an interesting analogy. The illegal immigration situation is somewhat like Prohibition. Americans tried to ban alcohol by constitutional amendment. It didn't work and was repealed. Instead alcohol was pretty well regulated by a variety of liquor laws. Similarly, Americans should now try to regulate illegal immigration.

So we have to deal with it, and that means some form of legalization. Moreover, three million children of illegals are legal U.S. citizens, born here. When they become adults they can take steps to legalize their illegal parents.

In the March/April 2004 edition of *Foreign Policy* magazine, some new logs were tossed onto the anti-immigration fire when Samuel Huntington published "The Hispanic Challenge," an excerpt from his new book *Who Are We?* In a harsh and unfair analysis, Huntington quotes a variety of Mexicans and Mexican Americans who wish to make the United States into a bilingual nation. Thus he reports that in 2003 more than 40 percent of the city of Hartford, Connecticut, is now made up of Hispanics, compared to 38 percent black. (He does not mention that the Hartford Metropolitan Statistical Area, which includes Hartford's suburbs, is 81 percent white.) He quotes Hartford's Hispanic-American mayor: "Hartford has become a Latin city, so to speak. It's a sign of things to come." And from Osvaldo Soto, president of the Spanish American League: "English is not enough. . . . We don't want a monolingual society."

Huntington also cites the "takeover" of the city of Miami by Cubans and notes that Cuban growth there has made Miami "an international economic dynamo, with expanding international trade and investment" leading to "dramatic personal income growth." That's bad?

But it's culture that seems to drive Huntington to distraction. He offers a 1995 quote from Jorge Castañeda, who later became Mexico's foreign minister: "Castañeda cited differences in social and economic quality, the unpredictability of events, concepts of time epitomized in the mañana syndrome, the ability to achieve results quickly, and attitudes toward history, expressed in the cliché that Mexicans are obsessed with history, Americans with the future." Huntington also offers the remarks of Lionel Sosa, a successful Mexican-American businessman, about "Hispanic traits" that "holds us Latinos back" in America: "mistrust of people outside of the family; lack of initiative, self-reliance and ambition; little use for education; and acceptance of poverty as a virtue necessary for entrance into heaven."

Huntington acknowledges that more than 90 percent of second- and third-generation Mexican Americans speak English well, but he finds it troubling that some of them learn Spanish as adults—as if learning French might be better.

In response, James Smith of the Rand Corporation suggested that "Huntington's analysis appeared not to distinguish fully between the experiences of first-generation immigrants and those of their children and grandchildren. . . . A more precise analysis would show that Hispanic immigrants have actually made rapid progress from generation to generation." Rodolfo O. De la Garza of Columbia University charged that "Huntington's fear that Hispanic immigrants would maintain strong loyalties to their countries of origin was not grounded in empirical fact." He cited research showing that Hispanic residents of the United States have a relatively low level of engagement with the policies of their home countries and are much more oriented to events in the United States.

In a letter to *Foreign Policy*, Andres Jiménez, director of the University of California's California Research Policy Center, cited research showing that Hispanic parents are more likely to attend PTA meetings and help their children with homework than are other Americans, and that Huntington's article was "misinformed, factually inaccurate, inflammatory, and potentially injurious to public policy because of its potential for being used as a baseless rationalization for anti-immigrant and anti-Mexican politics."

Huntington does not mention it, but it should be noted that there has been something of an explosion of interest in Hispanic music among young Americans. The artists include Enrique Iglesias, Jennifer

Lopez, Carlos Santana, Shakira, Gloria Estefan, Marc Anthony, Ricky Martin, and Christina Aguilera—some of Mexican descent, some not. Other Latins have entertained earlier generations of Americans— Linda Darnell, Ricardo Montalban, Desi Arnaz, Carmen Miranda, Anthony Quinn, and Rita Hayworth, to name a few.

No large immigration will be without problems. Mexican Americans have higher crime rates than the American average—but lower than the African-American rate. On the other hand, Mexican-American young people have high school dropout rates that are higher than blacks, though real progress is being made. The Urban Institute demographer Jeffrey Passel notes that in 1970 just 56 percent of Latino young people (18–24), including those born in Mexico, graduated from high school or went further educationally. Today the figure is 77 percent.

A survey taken by the Pew Hispanic Center in 2002 shows that among third-generation Hispanics, 50 percent speak only English, 49 percent are bilingual, and 1 percent are proficient only in Spanish. Pew senior researcher Richard Fry explains that the survey shows that of the 49 percent bilingual group, only 10 percent use more Spanish than English in the public sphere—for example in the workplace. Only at home, says Fry, do Latinos use Spanish to a significant degree, typically with parents or grandparents. One may assume that as Hispanics move to the fourth and fifth generations, the "English only" proportion will grow.

Depending on whether "Hispanic" or "Mexican" ancestry is measured, from 1989 to 1999 Latino family income has grown a little faster or a little slower than the American average, and slightly faster than the rate for all American whites.

Something of what bothers Huntington has happened before in America. Passel points out that at different moments in the nineteenth century, about 40 percent of the foreign-born in the United States were of German or Irish extraction, larger than the current Mexican proportion.

Put mildly, Huntington and I see this matter of immigration quite differently. If Hispanic growth, legal and illegal, were to continue indefinitely, his argument might be worth taking seriously. But the demographic outlook does not support that view. I doubt that part of

America will be taken over by Mexico. In their book *Remaking the American Mainstream*, Richard Alba and Victor Nee point out that once Mexican Americans have children, they tend to lose most contact with their old villages and develop deep roots in the United States. And University of Southern California professor Dowell Myers notes that 68 percent of Latinos who have been in America for thirty years own their own home—a figure identical to the American average, though native-born Americans tend to own their dwelling at an earlier age.

We return again to Benjamin Franklin, who in colonial times bemoaned of German immigrants that "few of their children know English." But we know now that their descendants do.

It is not a disaster, nine million people wanting to work hard in America. But the illegality is disturbing. The long-term solution involves both demographics and economics.

As noted earlier, the Mexican TFR has fallen rapidly and is believed to be near the replacement rate (notwithstanding the UN's 2.5 projected figure for 2000–2005). Jeffrey Passel notes that every year since 1990 the number of Mexican births has diminished and that this trend will continue as far as the statistical eye can see.

Couple that idea with another noted earlier: the Less Developed Countries are getting richer at a faster rate than the More Developed Countries.

So long term we will see a world whose population is shrinking and whose economic inequalities are slowly closing. That is not the recipe for an ongoing flood of illegal immigrants.

NO SENSE avoiding it. There can be real or perceived foreign policy problems with an immigrant nation. It is said that America often tilts to Greece, not Turkey, because America has a comparatively large and active Greek-American community. America, it is noted, tilts toward Israel because of a comparatively large Jewish population which is politically active and often involved in political fund-raising. When a mini-war erupted between the United Kingdom and Argentina, perhaps the United States helped the Brits because so many Americans are of British ancestry. After heavy political pressure from African-American legislators, the United States boycotted South

Africa in order to end apartheid. The "Captive Nations" resolutions, it has been maintained, were designed to mollify Americans of Eastern European descent. Now it is said that President Bush endorsed a new amnesty program to win the votes of Mexican Americans—and so on.

Should American foreign policy reflect the interest of Americans, or the American interest? It is a question without a good answer.

And yet Americans have managed rather well. They fought two twentieth-century wars against Germany despite a very large population of Americans of German descent. Italy was also an American enemy, although there is a very large population of Italo-Americans. And those so-called hyphenated Americans generally served in the American armed forces with distinction against their ancestral homelands. Americans have managed, and will continue to do so, case by case.

Other immigrant factoids:

*Immigrants are likely to live an average of three years longer than Americans born in America, according to a May 2004 National Institutes of Health study. The research, developed by Gopal K. Singh, shows that the largest gap is among native-born African Americans and foreign-born black Africans. The immigrants are likely to live nine years longer! How so? Lifestyle. Generally, immigrants drink less, are less obese, exercise more, and smoke less.

*Asian Indians are the second-largest legal immigrant group coming to America—1.65 million of them were enumerated in the 2000 Census. Their household median income was $63,699 per year, the highest of any ancestral group, probably settling a long-standing intuitive argument over whether Jews or Episcopalians are the wealthiest group in America. The Census Bureau doesn't measure by religion, hence there is no available data for Episcopalians, but the National Jewish Population Study of 2000 shows Jewish household income at $54,000, well below the Asian Indian figure.

*A variety of surveys show immigrants are somewhat more patriotic than the American average.

*In the long visa delays engendered by the effort to keep out terrorism, it has become harder to attract Muslim exchange students to America, which doesn't seem to be in the U.S. interest. America should keep up the scrutiny but accelerate the process.

*Immigrants in the United States and their children have often led the fight for liberty in their original home countries. They are often more famous in those nations than they are in the United States.

By and large, immigration has been good for America and will continue to be so. The goose lays good eggs.

Part Three

PROBLEMS, PRIDE, PERPLEXITY

An author tracing the spoor of an idea can become single-minded. I plead guilty. An article in the newspaper says we're killing too many whales. Don't worry, I say to myself, the demand situation may grow worse (as population grows from 6 billion to about 8 billion). It may grow still worse as populations get richer, that is, if they get richer and also enjoy eating whale meat. But then demand for whale meat will sink as population falls, probably well below 6 billion over a period of decades and centuries. The whales will be saved.

I have tried to sketch here a portrait of a very different world that is already coming upon us. I believe that America is the key actor in the New Demography. I believe that most of what I see America doing—growing, reproducing, standing up for political, social, and individual liberty, taking in immigrants—is beneficial, for us and for the rest of the world.

The New Demography will play a major role in global affairs in the decades to come. America is in comparatively good shape, but it is by no means immune from the demographic waves washing across the world nor the other problems that face mankind. We have problems that can match our pride if we are not alert.

CHAPTER THIRTEEN

Numbers Matter

THE UNITED NATIONS POPULATION DIVISION can appropriately brag about its own work as "momentous." The new numbers are amazing; this I knew when I started. But when I began this book I had no idea how wide its range would reach. Let me now review the major findings.

FIRST, the stunning new demographic facts are wholly unexpected. In both the More Developed Countries (mostly well-to-do and modern) and the Less Developed Countries (mostly poor, with some exceptions), the recent numbers are astonishing. Total Fertility Rates—the number of children born on average to women during their childbearing years—are falling dramatically almost everywhere.

Current global population should grow from about six billion to eight to nine billion, after which the United Nations Population Division projects a *decline*. That is the essence of the New Demography—what happens when a birth dearth follows a population explosion, with a longevity leap thrown in for good measure.

In the modern nations the TFRs have collapsed—America excepted. Most nations in Europe, and some other areas, are in panic. As recently as the 1985–1990 time frame, just fifteen years ago, the European TFR was 1.83 children per woman, within clear striking range of the "replacement" rate of 2.1. But now the European TFR is at 1.38 children per woman, a loss of close to half a child per

Countries with Below Replacement-Level Fertility in 2000–2005

Rank	MDC/LDC*	Region	Country Name	TFR, 2000–2005	Total Population (in 1,000), 2000
1	LDC	Asia	China, Hong Kong	1	6,807
2	LDC	Asia	China, Macao	1.1	450
3	MDC	Europe	Bulgaria	1.1	8,099
4	MDC	Europe	Latvia	1.1	2,373
5	MDC	Europe	Russian Federation	1.14	145,612
6	MDC	Europe	Slovenia	1.14	1,990
7	LDC	Asia	Armenia	1.15	3,112
8	MDC	Europe	Spain	1.15	40,752
9	MDC	Europe	Ukraine	1.15	49,688
10	MDC	Europe	Czech Republic	1.16	10,269
11	LDC	Asia	Republic of Korea	1.17**	46,835
12	MDC	Europe	Belarus	1.2	10,034
13	MDC	Europe	Hungary	1.2	10,012
14	MDC	Europe	Estonia	1.22	1,367
15	MDC	Europe	Italy	1.23	57,536
16	MDC	Europe	Lithuania	1.25	3,501
17	MDC	Europe	Poland	1.26	38,671
18	MDC	Europe	Greece	1.27	10,903
19	MDC	Europe	Austria	1.276	8,102
20	MDC	Europe	Slovakia	1.28	5,391
21	MDC	Europe	Bosnia and Herzegovina	1.3	3,977
22	MDC	Europe	Romania	1.32	22,480
23	MDC	Asia	Japan	1.32	127,034
24	MDC	Europe	Germany	1.35	82,282
25	LDC	Asia	Singapore	1.358	4,016
26	LDC	Asia	Georgia	1.4	5,262
27	MDC	Europe	Republic of Moldova	1.4	4,283
28	MDC	Europe	Switzerland	1.409	7,173
29	MDC	Europe	Portugal	1.45	10,016
30	MDC	North America	Canada	1.477	30,769
31	LDC	Latin America and Caribbean	Barbados	1.5	267
32	MDC	Europe	Channel Islands	1.54	144
33	LDC	Latin America and Caribbean	Cuba	1.55	11,202
34	LDC	Latin America and Caribbean	Trinidad and Tobago	1.55	1,289
35	MDC	Europe	United Kingdom	1.6	58,689
36	MDC	Europe	Sweden	1.635	8,856
37	MDC	Europe	Croatia	1.65	4,446
38	MDC	Europe	Serbia and Montenegro	1.65	10,555
39	MDC	Europe	Belgium	1.66	10,251
40	MDC	Oceania	Australia	1.696	19,153
41	MDC	Europe	Netherlands	1.72	15,898
42	MDC	Europe	Finland	1.73	5,177
43	MDC	Europe	Luxembourg	1.73	435
44	MDC	Europe	Malta	1.766	389
45	MDC	Europe	Denmark	1.77	5,322
46	MDC	Europe	Norway	1.795	4,473
47	LDC	Asia	China	1.825	1,275,215
48	MDC	Europe	France	1.89	59,296
49	LDC	Latin America and Caribbean	Puerto Rico	1.892	3,816
50	LDC	Latin America and Caribbean	Martinique	1.9	386
51	MDC	Europe	Ireland	1.9	3,819
52	MDC	Europe	Macedonia	1.9	2,024
53	LDC	Asia	Cyprus	1.903	783
54	LDC	Asia	Thailand	1.925	60,925
55	LDC	Africa	Mauritius	1.947	1,186
56	LDC	Asia	Kazakhstan	1.95	15,640
57	MDC	Europe	Iceland	1.952	282
58	LDC	Africa	Tunisia	2.006	9,519
59	LDC	Asia	Sri Lanka	2.008	18,595
60	MDC	Oceania	New Zealand	2.01	3,784
61	MDC	North America	United States	2.01†	290,809††
62	LDC	Asia	North Korea	2.021	22,268
63	LDC	Latin America and Caribbean	Netherlands Antilles	2.051	215

Source: United Nations Population Division, World Population Prospects: The 2002 Revision.

* MDC = More Developed Countries; LDC = Less Developed Countries
** Source: South Korean National Statistical Office, 2002
† Source: United States National Center for Health Statistics, 2002
†† Source: United States Census Bureau, 2003

woman in less than one generation. A similar situation obtains in Japan. There the TFR in the 1980–1985 time frame was 1.76 children per woman. In 2004 it was announced at 1.29 for 2003, down from 1.32, with the drop below 1.3 regarded by many Japanese officials as symbolically catastrophic. There are no indications that these rates will reverse themselves any time soon. They have been declining for more than four decades. It is not a blip.*

In 2002 the UN Population Division officially recognized these plummeting rates and keyed their official projections to 1.85 children per woman, for the first time a rate below the replacement level of 2.1. This was an act of belated bureaucratic and scientific courage that should now change the way we think.

Meanwhile, remarkably, the American TFR has risen. America now has the highest TFR of any major modern nation in the world. It was 1.92 children per woman in 1985–1990 and 2.01 in 2002. America will grow by at least 100 million people in the next 45 years while Europe loses about 100 million people and possibly more.

American growth will come about principally because of immigration. That roiling issue is likely to become even more intense here in the United States and particularly in Europe where the immigrants are mostly Muslims, at a time when the world is on edge due to terrorism perpetrated by fundamentalist Islamists. To be sure, the terrorists and their ardent sympathizers represent only a small minority of the Muslim population, but the terrorist threat is major and ongoing. Europeans had a great distaste for immigrants even before 9/11; since then it has grown.

What has happened demographically in the Less Developed Countries is perhaps still more remarkable. In the course of the past thirty-five years the Total Fertility Rate has plummeted from 6.01 children per woman to 2.92 in the 2000–2005 time frame. It is almost surely somewhat lower than that now—I'd put it about 2.7 or 2.8. The number of poor countries that have already fallen below

---

*Despite these trends, there is reason to expect human survival. Certain groups not only have high numbers of children but also believe in high fertility as an article of faith. These include the Mormons and Hutterites in the United States and ultra-Orthodox Jews in Israel and the United States. Even Mormons and Hutterites have experienced declines in TFRs although they remain above replacement.

replacement has climbed from sixteen to twenty in the last two years. Unofficially, still other countries have already crossed the replacement threshold, including some very big ones: Mexico, Brazil, and Iran. One official LDC, South Korea, has just reported an astonishing 2003 TFR of 1.17 children per woman, down from 1.41 the preceding year. That is lower than Italy's and those of some other European countries whose rates are in the cellar.

To explain why these rates have fallen, we look to some old correlations. These include increased contraception, the move from farm to city, education and work in the paid economy for women, legal abortion, divorce, the rising age of marriage ("fertility delayed is fertility denied"), the public emergence of the homosexual lifestyle, rising incomes, and the apparent separation of fertility decline from socio-economic gain—to begin a long list. Meanwhile, attempts at "pro-natalism," that is, efforts to increase fertility, have proven to be largely ineffective, and unaffordable in any event. Such efforts include child allowances, tax credits, day care, and paid parental leave.

The only apparent tendency in the other direction concerns new techniques for fertility enhancement. They have brought great joy to many parents, but the numbers involved are still so small as to have almost no impact on the larger demographic trends.

FALLING FERTILITY (along with rising life expectancy and rapidly aging populations) has caused serious pension and health-care problems. The problems are very large in the United States and monumental in Europe and Japan. The plausible remedies are either unpleasant or very unpleasant: taxes may be raised, or benefits cut, probably by raising the age of retirement. Some of the changes may occur in the United States fairly soon, at least if Alan Greenspan has anything to say about it. But the shortfalls in Europe are much greater. The estimated costs of fulfilling promises already made by government to voters are so large they cannot even be effectively measured, though they must be counted in the *quadrillions* of dollars. The titanic political battles we are now seeing are only the beginning.

On the upside there may be a *deus ex machina*. A significant boost in Gross Domestic Product rates, triggered by a new and better business climate, new science, and startling technology, could change the equation, possibly moving the aging/fertility situation from a "looming crisis" to an "ongoing problem." Economic growth is good; more growth is better.

Yet the coming commercial situation in Europe and Japan does not appear healthy, notwithstanding their high levels of technology and the beginnings of new economic regulations designed to accommodate the further growth of democratic capitalism. I find it unlikely that nations facing fewer births, fewer customers, and an aging problem will show substantial economic growth rates.

THERE IS A commercial point here that should be of particular interest to those in and around the business community. Beyond TFRs, I have emphasized evidence that the poor countries (LDCs) are moving ahead economically more rapidly than the modern countries. This is a new world: poor countries with low and falling fertility rates are growing wealthier faster than rich modern countries. These facts produce some dazzling patterns.

Globally, the biggest economic news concerns India, which in fiscal year 2003 grew by 8.1 percent, a rate which the World Bank and many financial analysts and economists believe will continue at a high level for a good while. Some of the recent Indian growth has been due to particularly good farming weather. On the other hand, a modernizing India depends less on agricultural exports than previously. Even should the monsoons fail to continue their good run, India's progress represents a large step toward boosting the sluggish world economy.

Altogether, the Less Developed Countries face a potentially beneficial "demographic dividend." Because their TFRs were so high a generation ago, they now have a huge cohort of potential young workers. (There are 537 million people under age 24 in India alone.) These young LDC workers are better educated than their parents, have fewer children, have more money per person to spend, and—still the key comparative advantage—work for relatively cheap wages, sometimes very cheap. (But time marches on. With Indian income on the rise, some Indian economists are now concerned that foreign firms invested in India will soon be looking for economic platforms with wage scales even lower than India's.)

India already has 1.1 billion people and is projected to grow to about 1.5 billion before beginning to decline. China (population 1.3 billion) is expected to top out at 1.4 billion people and has enjoyed stellar economic growth rates in the annual range of 7 to 9 percent. These two billionaire nations, with the United States, are likely to be the logical new "locomotive" economies of the years to come. India and China each have many problems, however, and will bear close scrutiny. Some geopolitical professionals claim that one or both will "break apart," potentially causing major economic turmoil. I doubt this will happen in India; it is a democratic nation, and that plays a crucial role in its unity. China, as a nondemocratic nation, has a situation more difficult to predict.

Beyond the demographic dividend, the LDC nations are harnessing the forces of science and technology and beginning to marry them to the commercial creativity of market capitalism, yielding a brighter global economic situation.

While India is the most spectacular global economic story at the moment, from a U.S. point of view what is happening in Mexico is probably more important. According to the country's leading demographers, the TFR in Mexico is already at or below the replacement rate. In coming decades this trend, coupled with decent economic growth, may substantially change immigration patterns into the United States, both legal and illegal. The turmoil caused by illegal immigration to the United States is probably not a condition that will continue forever.

THE COMING OF THE NEW DEMOGRAPHY plays a fascinating role within the environmental community. Many activist environmentalists believe that our human problem is *too many people*, particularly wealthy, polluting types with their SUVs and sprawling, energy-consuming houses. They fear that humanity is growing on automatic pilot. So they argue that as America grows by at least 100 million people, pollution will worsen. They demand we invest in their favorite remedies. This idea animates the global warming debate.

The facts seem to play out differently. An examination of pollution rates in the modern affluent countries in recent decades shows a great improvement. In America this is clearly demonstrated by data published by the Environmental Protection Agency. In almost every measurable way in the United States, notwithstanding major population growth, the environment is getting better. The same pattern holds true in most other modern nations. It surely seems that more well-to-do people do not cause more pollution, if those people set their mind to seeing that it does not happen.

THE GEOPOLITICAL EFFECTS of falling fertility are likely to be vast. Population has an effect on power and gross economic potency. As it loses 100 million people, Europe will likely have even less relative power in the years to come. That may mean that America must shoulder more of the load in defending and promoting the values of Western civilization. But Europe should not be written off easily. In 2050 there will still be more Europeans than Americans, and it is a well-to-do continent. Still, it will experience significant depopulation, not a sign associated with military might.

Military power is related to population. In its simplest formulation, defense costs a great deal of money. But it is mostly a fixed cost. Thus a nation with a growing population—like America—can fund a powerful and growing military without tax increases, or at least not heavy ones. The military fixed costs will be divided among more taxpayers. The reverse is true in Europe and Japan.

Beyond military power, I take it as the American mission to promote the global growth of individual and economic liberty within a democratic context. Recent data show a stunning worldwide growth in such liberties, despite periodic setbacks in individual nations. In a world where the big new population numbers are coming from the Less Developed Countries, they need our help.

For both these tasks, America has the wallet, but does it have the will? I believe it does, with either a Republican or a Democrat in the White House, with either Republican or Democratic majorities in Congress.

Once again India may be a critical indicator, precisely because it is not a new democracy. Its representative government, while not perfect, goes back half a century. That gives the lie to the idea that advanced forms of democratic governments are only for well-to-do nations. India has been poor and democratic. Within two or three decades it may well be middle class and democratic.

The continued promotion of democracy may well be the best way to fight global terrorism. People who run their own countries don't like it when those countries are blown up, whether in Washington, Madrid, or Baghdad. Without a prospering and demographically growing example of liberty—America—it would be harder to pursue the continuing growth of liberty. A very old human dream, liberty is only now reaching global fruition. Democracy cannot be imposed, but it can be encouraged.

For many years there was a struggle within the American foreign policy community between the pragmatic "realists" and the starry-eyed "idealists." In a series of major speeches, President George W. Bush settled the argument, at least for now. America will be the enthusiastic leader in the struggle for global democratic governance. Such a view now represents more than just the preachments of neoconservative and other human rights groups and some active supply-side theoreticians. It is the stated policy of the government of the United States of America. It would be very hard to reverse, assuming any new president really wanted to do so.

I do not believe it is an accident that the one area in the world without any democratic states is precisely the source of the principal terrorists: the Arab world. That is one reason why the struggle to establish a representative government in Iraq is so important.

THE PROBLEMS brought about by immigration are enormous and promise to grow. Only 3 percent of the global population are immigrants, but they constitute far more than 3 percent of the world's problems. Two issues stand out, intertwined: illegality and distaste. It has proved next to impossible to stop poor people—the great majority of them young adults—from moving to well-to-do countries where they can better themselves and their families.

In America the most publicized immigration issue concerns Mexicans. This is true notwithstanding the fact that Mexican Americans are assimilating into the American mainstream economically and, most important, culturally. A recent book by Samuel Huntington, *Who Are We?*, raises fears of a bilingual America. I do not go to sleep worrying about it. It is hard for me to visualize a world that is "Americanizing" while America is "Mexicanizing."

The anti-Mexican feeling in America is gentle compared with anti-immigrant attitudes in Europe, where immigrants come mostly from the Arab countries and Muslim Turkey (to Germany). "Hatred" may not be too strong a word.

The European nations, unlike America, are not at root pluralist and their citizens do not like it when others butt in. The formation of the European Union was supposed to create a new sense of Europeanism, with open borders among its members. Perhaps some day. But today many citizens of "Old Europe" are complaining about Poles, Hungarians, Bulgarians, and other Eastern Europeans willing to work for low wages and taking up residence in the wealthier high-welfare societies of the West.

The UN's numbers in this book include both legal immigrants and estimates for illegal immigrants. In Europe the arriving immigrants, of both sorts, are principally from North Africa, the Middle East, and Turkey. Accordingly, demographic and ethnic balance in Europe is changing. One estimate is that 20 to 24 million Muslims are already in Europe, and the number is growing. A popular estimate claims that 25 percent of French schoolchildren are of Muslim ancestry. Another back-of-the-envelope estimate puts the number of Arabs in Italy, Spain, and France—old Europe—growing to more than a third of working adults. Mosques seem to rise almost everywhere on the continent. Moreover the Total Fertility Rate of Muslims is apparently somewhat higher than that of the European countries in which they reside, although good data is hard to come by.

The Ottoman Suleiman the Magnificent reached the gates of Vienna before he was turned back. Today Europe has become mostly secular, and immigration has come principally from nonsecular Arab nations. In a recent article the historian Niall Ferguson speculates that one European scenario foresees a "creeping Islamicization of a decadent Christendom." The title of Ferguson's article was "Eurabia." In the decades to come we may witness great ethnic change in anti-pluralist and shrinking Europe. This process may be peaceful or not. Meanwhile, an optimistic America that has accommodated pluralism will be growing substantially in the years ahead.

I HAVE frequently used the phrase "America excepted" in this book. Indeed America has the highest Total Fertility Rate among the major modern nations. American population will grow substantially while others shrink. America is the richest and most powerful nation in the world, and is likely to remain so. It is good that Americans are optimistic and believe their country stands for something unique in the world, which deserves to be promoted. It is good that transnational polls show Americans as the world's most patriotic people, and that Americans believe theirs is a work in progress. It is heartening to see in those polls that immigrants to America are even more patriotic than other Americans. It is good that American taxpayers are prepared to pay for a mighty military. But Americans also have their own plateful of problems related to demographics.

One of the great buzzwords of our time is "multi-culturalism." In one sense it is used to describe the pluralism of a nation united by the gradual blending of immigrants. In *The First Universal Nation*, I argued that America was the first nation where people came from everywhere else, and that was the source of our greatest strength. America, I maintained, was a mostly tolerant place.

In 1999 the distinguished political scientist Alan Wolfe and a team of researchers interviewed two hundred middle-class suburbanites across America for his book *One Nation, After All*.* Wolfe told me: "With the exception of the issue of homosexuality, the change in American public opinion toward greater tolerance in the past few decades has been truly remarkable. And in the five years since publication of the book there is evidence of more tolerance on the homosexuality issue."

In early 2004, Henry Kissinger remarked in an interview: "There's no country that you can come to as a fifteen-year-old, speak all your life with an accent, become secretary of state during a period when the president is under siege, and have almost presidential powers. And while I got many nasty letters, I never got a letter saying, 'Who are you to be in this position?' That couldn't happen anywhere else. . . ."

That's one kind of multi-culturalism. On the other hand, and greatly disturbing, is the multi-culturalism that has become the rally-

---

*The respondents came from eight suburbs: Brookline and Medford, Massachusetts; Southeast DeKalb County and Cobb County, Georgia; Broken Arrow and Sand Springs, Oklahoma; Eastlake and Rancho Bernardo, California.

ing cry for those who prefer separatism and like to talk about the "American peoples" (plural *s*). They seek an America divided by race, ethnicity, gender, sexual preference, class, and language. They push for quotas in hiring and in school admissions (admittedly a much more complex issue). They want Americans considered as groups, not as individuals.

This line is espoused by relatively few activists, but it receives a wide hearing among the babbling bunches, often in the academic world. They attempt to influence students* and gain considerable media coverage. The separatists set up a model that says America has two groups, the oppressed and the oppressors.

This is separatism with a purpose, espoused by those—mostly on the left, but some on the right—who believe that America needs a radical transformation. This kind of social fragmentation could be highly injurious to the continued success of the United States. It scorns patriotism; it is sometimes called "post-patriotic." Too often it seeks to use a generally healthy immigration to turn America inward against itself. It could make a strong, diverse, and growing America into a weakened target to those who wish us ill, in a time of global terrorism. It is disuniting at a time when we need all the unity we can get.

Most observers, on all points on the political spectrum, agree that Americans don't know much about the country of which they are so proud. A 2000 survey by the American Council of Trustees and Alumni showed that among seniors in the fifty-five most elite colleges and universities in America, 81 percent were graded F or D after taking a test based on American history questions from a typical *high school* curriculum. No wonder: not a single one of those "best" institutions of higher learning required a course in American history. Not one.

---

*Anecdotal reports indicate that college students these days are more moderate and conservative than they used to be, and less liberal than their 1960s-activated faculties in the humanities departments. In 1970, among incoming freshmen, 45 percent characterized themselves as "middle of the road" and 17 percent as "conservative." In 2002 the middle-of-the-road figure climbed to 51 percent, and the conservative number rose slightly to 20 percent. (American Council on Education). I have been unable to find the self-identification of seniors.

Yes, American history is taught in our elementary schools, junior high schools, and high schools. But, as Churchill said, the pudding has no theme. In 2000, in its report "History Textbooks at the New Century," the American Textbook Council declared, "Faith in progress and patriotic pride have vanished. . . . What has replaced them is too often a nation that has repeatedly fallen short of its ideals, led by a patriarchy that deserves censure. . . ."

At issue is an elemental question: What will our children be taught? Should the American story be told to American children as value-neutral, with lots of guilt and atonement on display? Or should American children understand that their country has changed the world for the better in ways that matter the most.

Western civilization, of which America is now the point of the lance, is up against a ferocious enemy: Islamists who seek to destroy the modern and mostly beneficial American values that have shaped the modern world. Do not fool yourself: we do not know what the outcome of this struggle will be.

In October 1942, Thornton Wilder's play *The Skin of Our Teeth* was produced as the Nazis and Japanese moved toward global conquest. Wilder's notion was that Western civilization had been threatened before and had pulled through by the skin of its teeth. The historian Robert Conquest writes that the survival of Western civilization was "a near thing" during the years of the cold war. Today Islamist terrorists strike most everywhere. Even when they are foiled, it costs us, as when airline flights are canceled for fear of a terrorist strike. The mass bombing of the Madrid commuter trains in March 2004 apparently turned the Spanish national elections into a surprising upset victory for the Socialists.

If we want our coming generations to be strong in the parlous geopolitical days ahead they should know what the great contest is about. The American story is a great one, and understanding it accurately would make us stronger.

Americans believe in America. And Americans don't believe in ignorance. A recent survey commissioned by Public Agenda showed that 84 percent of parents believe that America is "a unique country that stands for something special in the world"—and they want that taught to their children. The same survey asked parents about race in

America: 89 percent of all parents, 88 percent of African Americans, and 84 percent of Hispanics believe "there's too much attention paid these days to what separates different ethnic and racial groups and not enough to what they have in common."

Low fertility has a profound personal effect on many individual Americans. Data from the 2002 Census Bureau Current Population Survey show a TFR for Americans born in America of 1.86 children per woman, for white non-Hispanics of 1.79, for Asian Americans of 1.62, for blacks of 1.94.* Beyond that, remember that low fertility also correlates with higher income, higher education, urban residence, and a woman's age, which would further lower these numbers for those persons who fall in those categories.

In thinking about this information, visualize some people you know. Think about your friend Amanda, the woman in the ad agency who delayed having children, then delayed further because she was getting a good promotion. Think about your friends Chris and Jennifer who have been divorced once, twice, or more, thus reducing the fertility rate. It is easy to see the demographic problems in Europe and Japan, but it's happening to some people in America too. Remember that 16 percent of American women ended up with no children in 2003, up from 11 percent in the early 1970s.

IF LOW FERTILITY PERSISTS in many modern countries, the human mind-set is fair game for change. It is not a new thing to be concerned about "an only child." Perhaps since the beginning of humankind, it has been claimed such children are more likely to be "spoiled." If so, we are likely in for more of that. As noted, a one-child family creates an arena where children grow up without brothers, sisters, uncles, aunts, cousins, and with as many as fourteen parents, grandparents, and great-grandparents (assuming rising life expectancies). In a one-child family, the child's only direct relatives are all ancestors.

Would all that change the nature of our behavior? It might. For one thing, parents with one child might not allow their child to take

---

*TFR data calculated by Martin O'Connell, chief, Fertility and Family Statistics Branch, U.S. Census Bureau.

the reasonable risks linked to learning about the world. They might be less willing to let their child join the military, even when necessary.

In certain areas of the less developed world, Asia particularly, sex-selected abortion has become commonplace where there is a powerful cultural preference for sons. What nature gives us from the womb is about 105 boy babies for every 100 girl babies. But traveling sonogram teams tell women the sex of their child in advance, and many females are aborted. In China the boy-girl ratio was 118 to 100 in the year 2000. In India it has climbed but not as high.

Thus in China there will likely be 10 to 15 percent "unmarriageable" men in the decades to come. This may improve the global condition of women.

The emeritus clinical psychologist David Gutmann of Northwestern notes that "Social mobility and urban society tend to demobilize the extended family—the major support system for parenthood, and especially motherhood. When the burdens of childrearing are shared out among sisters, cousins, aunts, mothers, and grandmothers, parenthood becomes more a joy than a burden, and is easily accepted. But childrearing in the unbuffered nuclear family, relatively isolated in the city . . . is very burdensome."

We may well see a lonelier world. Will "friends" become "like family"? Well, think of yourself in an assisted-living home. (The insurance companies selling long-term care policies say that 44 percent of seniors end up there.) And when that one child becomes an adult, she or he may be caught in the "sandwich trap," supporting college-age children while taking care of parents. Clergymen say the most sorrowful funerals are those in which the deceased has no children. And there is a "grandchild gap." People well into their sixties, seventies, or eighties are looking for grandchildren to love. Without them they can become deeply disappointed, even misanthropic.

And there is love. As an often-libertarian type, I approve of people having just as many children as they choose. But my own belief is that having and raising children is the essence of the human experience.

IN SUM, is this New Demography good or bad for humanity? It should be very good for the Less Developed Countries for at least several decades. At the same time it may be a disturbing mess for the modern nations of Europe and Japan, once major economic powers.

For those who say it is a good thing, the best answers concern demographic history. The optimists note that most every country and region has more population today than it had a hundred years ago, including Europe and Japan where population numbers are now fading. And they note that the world has generally improved.

Pessimists use the flip side of the same historical facts. What was so terrible about the 2.5 billion people of 1950 (when the current series of UN population data begins)? That was enough people to create an abundance of beneficial devices and procedures for the betterment of humankind.

It would not seem to be a big loss that we will never know, or never see, nor will our grandchildren or great-grandchildren ever know or see, what a world of twelve, fifteen, or twenty billion people would be like, though such allegedly expert projections were tossed around loosely only a few decades ago. To the contrary, the children of people alive today, or their children or grandchildren, may see a world of four billion people or fewer. In itself it is not a problem if populations decline, though the current speed of the decline may cause great problems.

WHY ARE fertility rates falling? Has secularization trumped religion? Is advancing materialism corroding our faith? Are we victims of too much freedom? Are we witnessing cultural decline? Are we committing environmental sins? There are many answers coming from many points on the spectrum.

I've asked these questions of people whom I respect, mostly Americans. Some say indeed it relates to the decline of religion—the Bible says, "Be fruitful, multiply, and replenish the earth." Others point to the new ability of women to work in the money economy—often a sound economic choice. Environmentalists think it's a good thing.

I have also talked recently to some young folks who are making these decisions about children, at least those relatively well-to-do Americans in urban settings. "The thirties today are what the twenties used to be," they say. "What's wrong with adopting when there are so many children in need?" "Have one, adopt one." "It's a limitation on personal freedom." "It's harder to have children the older you get, and women in their thirties are worried." "Men respond to cultural signals; sexual freedom and contraception have changed things." "Not a big deal if you don't have children." "It's so expensive."

Consider this: *In the modern countries, if nothing happens, something happens.* Is it irresponsible for the species to breed itself downward? Human life has a purpose. Human beings may choose not to have children, or to have only one child, but the human species does not have that choice. Yet the UN data points in that direction.

I have been called "a perpetual optimist." I have always preferred "realist." I think I've been an optimistic realist. But how does an optimistic realist deal with this February 2004 article in the newspaper *The Scotsman*: "The population of Scotland will fall below five million by 2009. . . . More worrying than the fact that the population is getting smaller is that it's also getting older as the birthrate falls significantly. All this suggests that by the year 3573 there'll be two people left in Scotland, probably a married couple in their 90s living in Beardsden." I don't know where Beardsden is, but I know that something strange and unnatural is happening.

People whom I talk with about these trends typically respond, "I had no idea." No excuses now.

Acknowledgments

FIRST THANKS go to my home base, the American Enterprise Institute. For a freelance fellow like myself, it has been like going to heaven. The AEI philosophy, near as I can figure out, is elemental: find the best people and leave them alone to do what they think is important. They will work harder that way. Elaborate staff meetings, hierarchies, and backbiting have simply not been part of my experience there.

AEI's president, Chris DeMuth, is a rare fellow: a first-class intellectual with great practical ability. That is a marvelous combination for a man to run a think tank like AEI. For almost twenty years he has given me sage advice and backed me up every step of the way. AEI's executive vice president, David Gerson, has always helped me when I needed help.

Others at AEI offered very specific assistance and are cited in the book: Joe Antos, Leon Aron, Karlyn Bowman, Nick Eberstadt, Eric Engen, Steve Hayward, and Josh Muravchik.

We have a lunchtime round table at AEI where a fellow can learn a great deal. I learned a lot there, and from other AEI colleagues. Among my tutors and helpers on various aspects of this book were John Lott, Gautam Adhikari, Bob Helms, Radek Sikorski, Marvin Kosters, Kevin Hassett, Jagadeesh Gokhale, Claude Barfield, Monty Brown, Veronique Rodman, Virginia Bryant, Karl Zinsmeister, Michael Novak, and Gene Hosey.

Research assistants Vance Serchuk, Anne Moore, Christina Imholt, Sean Gupta, Nell Manning, and Sharon Utz helped out regularly. Scott Palmer was of aid.

I'm not at all sure that AEI could run without Doris Gibson. This book could not have been written without the help of AEI's Robert Riley, who kept fixing my electronic hardware in times of crisis.

My research assistant at AEI is Jeremy Kadden. He is a very able young man with, I'm sure, a brilliant future. He worked long and hard on this project, and became somewhat of a demographic and economic maven. Not only that, he is a very nice person. And so are Todd Weiner and Hans Allhoff who worked on the early parts of the research. Bryan O'Keefe pulled a valuable oar at the final stage.

The second set of acknowledgments go to the United Nations Population Division, without whose help, rather obviously, this book could not have been written. The UNPD is professionally staffed by first-rate demographers who have been enormously helpful, prompt, and cordial. The UNPD director, Joseph Chamie, is a superb demographer and author. He has one of the great demographic stories ever on his hands, and he is trying to tell the world about it in both standard and original ways, with some real success. Here are some of the key players, alphabetically, who provided me with great help at the UNPD: Thomas Buettner, chief, Population Estimates and Projections Section; Joseph Grinblat, chief, Mortality and Migration Section; Larry Heligman, assistant director, Population Division; Sabine Henning, population affairs officer; Serguey Ivanov, population affairs officer; Vasantha Kandiah, chief, Fertility and Family Planning Section; Clare Menozzi, associate statistician, Demographic and Social Statistics Branch; Barry Mirkin, chief, Population Policy Section; Cheryl Sawyer, population affairs officer; Mary Beth Weinberger, chief, Population and Development Section; Hania Zlotnik, assistant director, Population Division.

The demographers and experts I sat with at several meetings hosted by the UNPD were of great help as are those who over the years I have learned from. There have been many; a few come to mind: Paul Demeny, John Bongaarts, Stephen Sindig, Samuel Preston, Jean-Claude Chenais, the late Egon Mayer, Sidney Goldstein, Charles Westhoff, and Richard Easterlin make the short list.

The statistical product of the United States government never fails to astonish me. They seem to have something about everything. As always, I owe a debt of thanks to the United States Census Bureau. It collects and publishes international as well as domestic data. Of particular help were Peter Way, John Long, Daniel Goodkind, Martin O'Connell, Tom McDevitt, and Dwight Johnson. At the National Center for Health Statistics I owe particular thanks to Stephanie Ventura, who has been helping me on matters statistical for quite some time now.

Thanks go to Penn Kemble, Carl Gershman, Cindy Balmuth, Ken Tomlinson, Robert Wright, Jonathan Schull, Sam Vaughan, David Kusnet, David Hendin, Michael Newman, Andy Walworth, John Sorensen, Candace Crandall, and Richard Alba. The following people helped either Jeremy or me, or both: Sumitra Chowdhury of the Indian embassy, Daniel Necas of the University of Minnesota, Chad Kolton at the Office of Management and Budget, Stan Henshaw and Rebecca Wind at the Alan Guttmacher Institute, Bill McCormick at the United States Agency for International Development, Gil Sewall at the American Textbook Council, Linda Chavez of the Center for Equal Opportunity, Andrew Biggs of the Cato Institute, Carl Haub of the Population Reference Bureau, Robert Leiken of the Nixon Center, Fred Singer of the Science and Environmental Policy Project, Michele Tribalat of the Institute National d'Etudes Demographiques, Tamar Jacoby of the Manhattan Institute, Anne Gauthier of the University of Calgary, and Lynn Tramonte of the National Immigration Forum.

My fine friend Judy Hanauer read the manuscript, provided useful comments, and kept me in receipt of a stream of relevant articles from all over the internet that show up in many places in this book.

Books don't get published without publishers, editors, and agents. This one was published by Ivan R. Dee, and Ivan also did the exceptional editing job on a complex book, replete with many charts. Special thanks too to Hilary Meyer, Joyce Marcum, and Judith Kelly at the Dee firm. My agent is Rafe Sagalyn, and I owe him a debt of thanks for his thoughtful and diligent work.

My children—in reverse chronological order, Rachel, Sarah, Daniel, and Ruth—helped me as they always have. My grandchildren are acknowledged in the dedication. Children and grandchildren are at the essence of demography.

Index

25, 67–82, 70, 71, 73–76, 78–79,
157, 174, 176, 191–205, 211,
216–217; Iraqi war, 181–182, 190;
Jewish community, 52n, 81; liberty
promotion, 158–159, 171–174, 175,
182–190, 207, 215; medical care,
125–127; military power, 10, 158,
168–169, 170–171, 176, 179;
minority classifications, 73; mobility
of population, 156; morale, 163–164;
multiculturalism, 70, 71, 218–219;
New Demography and, 7–8; pollution
levels, 154, 214; population, 5, 12,
26, 61–62, 75, 136, 155–157,
161–162, 167, 175, 197, 211;
problems, 207; Protestant TFR,
47–48; race distinctions, 18, 65, 66,
72–76, 220–221; racism, 68–69;
retirement age, 122; retirement plans,
119–121, 124, 128–133, 212;
separatism, 218–219; student political
leanings, 219, 219n; Total Fertility
Rates, 20–22, 24, 25, 26, 47–48, 52n,
61, 62–66, 65, 74n, 211, 221; UN
classification, 20, 60–62; urban
population, 94; Vietnam War,
163–164; White community TFR, 65
United States Information Agency
(USIA), 189
UNPD. *See* UN Population Division
Uprooted, The (Handlin), 69
Urban populations, 94–95, 94n, 95, 198
Uruguay, Total Fertility Rates, 49
USIA (United States Information
Agency), 189
USS Enterprise, 168

Vaesson, Martin, 113
Van de Kaa, D.J., 109
Vietnam, Total Fertility Rates, 56
Vietnam War, 163–164
Vietnamese immigrants, assimilation in
U.S., 70, 71
Vogel, Ezra, 178

Walker, Francis, 69
Wars: Arab/Israeli, 173; cold war, 172,
172n, 186–187; democracy and, 173,
173n, 179; fertility geared toward,
159–160; Total Fertility Rates affected
by, 21–22, 51, 56, 165, 167; U.S./Iraqi,
181–182, 190; Vietnam War, 163–164;
Western civilization and, 162; World
War II, 21–22, 165, 167, 186. *See also*
Military power; Terrorism.
Water pollution, 154
Watson Wyatt Worldwide, 116, 122
Wattenberg, Ben J.: TV interviews by,
32–33; TV interviews of, 78–79;
writing of, 10–11, 16, 79, 218. *See
also Birth Dearth.*
Western civilization, 160–171, 161,
173, 185–190, 220. *See also countries
by name.*
White TFR, United States, 65
Who Are We? (Huntington), 201–204,
216
Wilder, Thornton, 220
Williamson, Jeffrey, 196
Winter, Jay, 17, 159n
Wolfe, Alan, 218
Women: education and its effects, 95–96,
96, 97; paid labor and fertility rates, 96
World Bank, economic projections,
143–144
"World Population in 2300" (UNPD),
147
World Population Prospects (UN),
11–12, 11n, 26, 54, 83
World War II: alternate outcomes, 186;
fertility rates affected by, 21–22, 165,
167
Worldwatch Institute, 152–153

Young, Whitney, 194
Yoshiro Mori, 133n

Zakaria, Fareed, 189
Zangwill, Israel, 80

A NOTE ON THE AUTHOR

Ben J. Wattenberg is a Senior Fellow at the American Enterprise Institute in Washington, D.C. For the past eleven years he has moderated the prize-winning weekly PBS television discussion program "Think Tank with Ben Wattenberg." He has written ten books, many of which have shaped the public dialogue, including *Values Matter Most*; *The Real Majority* and *The Real America* (with Richard Scammon); *The Birth Dearth*; and *The Good News Is the Bad News Is Wrong*. Mr. Wattenberg worked as a speechwriter for President Lyndon B. Johnson as well as in campaigns for Senator Henry "Scoop" Jackson and Senator Hubert Humphrey. He was a member of the U.S. delegation to the 1984 UN World Population Conference and has participated in population symposia with the UN Population Division, the National Academy of Science, the Population Association of America, and the American Association for the Advancement of Science. He lives in Washington, D.C.